THE LOST LIFE

OF

TILLY MACLEOD

A. L. DOWIE

Published by L J Legg
1 High Street
Hope Valley S32 4TL

A paperback original 2024

First published in Great Britain by L J Legg 2024
As part of a wide-ranging, fundraising and awareness project for dementia.

Copyright © L J Legg writing as A. L. Dowie 2024

The moral right of L J Legg writing as A.L. Dowie to be identified as the author of this work has been asserted in accordance with the Copyright, Designs and Patents Act of 1988.

A CIP catalogue record for this book is available from the British Library.

ISBN: 978 1 0687124 0 1

This novel is entirely a work of fiction. The names, characters and incidents portrayed in it are the work of the author's imagination or are used fictitiously. Any resemblance to actual persons, living or dead, is entirely coincidental.

All rights reserved. No part of this publication may be reproduced, stored in a retrieval system, or transmitted, in any form or by any means, electronic, mechanical, photocopying, recording or otherwise, without prior permission of the publisher.

Printed and bound by
Swallowtail Print,
Drayton Industrial Park, Taverham Road,
Drayton, Norwich, Norfolk. NR8 6RL

I have had the honour to know many wonderful people who in the final years of their lives, had to face one of the biggest challenges a human-being can experience. A life with dementia.

Each person kept so much of their individuality through to the end, whilst simultaneously losing almost everything we had known them to be.

Gradually losing each of these people, drew my attention to how families and social groups construct themselves around their beliefs about individual members and the role that each person performs within the group. Each loss also changed my understanding of myself.

This book is dedicated to all individuals and families living with dementia.

This copy has been created by the author as part of a fundraising and awareness campaign for dementia. Please pass it on, or donate it to charity, to help keep dementia support a topic of conversation.

Prologue

Isla - 2024

I look down at the letter in my hands. Although the original version wasn't sent to me, this short communication had the unexpected power to utterly transform my life, and my sense of self. Quite something for such an insubstantial document. It's no more than a few heartfelt words and could so easily have been dismissed as insignificant, because my mother chose never to respond.

Dearest one,
I worry about you starting your new life with James without us all around.
I know that I will never understand the pain that you carry, and it is clear, that in your mind, the only way to cope is with a completely fresh start.
Please know that we are here, waiting with open arms should you feel able to return.
In the meantime, I wish you joy and above all else, security. James is a good man. He has proven himself and he will look after you. - Trust him!
Your ever-loving,
Simone

One

Isla - 2015

I adore this moment when the train finally pulls into the station in West Kilbride. I'm home. I get a warm, fuzzy feeling every time I arrive, even though it's more than thirty years since I lived here.

The flowers in the hanging baskets, the wood-panelled seating area on the single platform with the row of hills in the distance down the line, all call out to my teenage self.

The day that Mam agreed I could travel without her on this line was the day that I embraced the wider world and started to question my place within it.

I'm meeting Mam and Da in *The Glen* for fish and chips. The ones from the shop are no match for what Mam produced when Da brought the fish home, but they stay a favourite meal, because we always eat them outdoors.

They've become a tradition on my visits home, as the trains from the airport aren't always on time. I glance at my watch. Only ten minutes late today. I pull my document bag from the shelf overhead and head to my suitcase, which is lodged beside the central doors. It's a beautiful evening, and my stomach is rumbling.

I'm attracting a few prolonged looks. I'm not the only person on the train in office wear, but I'm the smartest dressed by far, and my document bag and suitcase set me apart from the tourists travelling with their backpacks.

I make quite a noise as I head along the street. The clack of my heels competes with the relentless trundle of my suitcase. Da has heard me coming and is hurrying towards me as I enter *The Glen*, arms wide open.

I stand for a moment, wrapped in his embrace.

I may oversee the whole European division at work, but there is nothing better than knowing I can return to my father's arms and feel small, carefree, and protected every now and again.

He picks up my suitcase and we walk down the path to join Mam. She doesn't get up, but raises her arms to me, and I slide onto the bench beside her so that we can hug.

I'm shocked to feel her ribs beneath my hands. She's lost a lot of weight since I was here last.

'Hi Mam, you ok?' I ask a little too brightly.

Mam seems distracted by a toddler, playing on the grass with a large beach ball. I can't get her to look at me.

It's a new response, but I'm used to the initial unease between us when I first arrive. I'm rarely here longer than a day or two, but we usually stop circling each other like a pair of leopards long before it's time for me to head home. Back to my other home that is. Dortmund.

Da reaches into the insulated bag that's waiting in the centre of the blanket which they've brought for me, so that we don't have to sit on the bench in a long line. He brings out two neatly wrapped parcels. Small haddock and chips for me, and a large cod and chips for them to share. The order never changes.

As he hands me my packet, he asks in an undertone so that Mam can't hear.

'How're things in Germany?'

Taking care to use an equally quiet voice I reply,

'I've been given the go ahead to draw up a plan for an international merger. If I can attract interest from the right company, it could save my division.'

'Good on you girl!' He whispers quietly, lightly punching my arm as he turns to stand up.

I glance up at Mam and relax. She hasn't noticed.

Da, meanwhile, has crossed to the bench and hands her their meal to unwrap.

I appreciate that he continues to risk upsetting Mam by asking about my life in Dortmund.

Mam made it clear many years ago that if I went to work overseas, she didn't want to hear anything about my life there, and she has stuck vehemently to this position for three decades.

This of course leaves me in a familiarly impossible position. My whole life is wrapped up in my work in Dortmund, so I have little else to talk about. In the end, as I settle on the blanket and unwrap my fish, I resort to a tried and tested topic.

'So Da, what news from the golf club?'

Isla - 2015

I look down at my mud-caked walking boots as the train pulls into the station. I look a little different from yesterday. I wonder if there's anyone here to make the comparison.

Da has gone quiet again. It happened a few times during our walk and each of those times I put it down to climbing a particularly steep incline, or getting lost in the view, but this is not like him. We are usually so happy to see each other that we can't stop talking.

As we step from the train, I take hold of his elbow and pull him to a standstill.

'Da, what's the matter? You've got something on your mind.'

'Nothing for you to worry about Isla. Have you a few more steps in you? Or do you want to take a bus to The Hydro? I told your mother we'd meet her there in half an hour.'

'I'm fine to walk, although I can't be sure that my boots can say the same. Look at them! The stitching is all coming undone and the soles have almost no grip left. I almost came a cropper on that scree section this morning.'

'They've done you well.' He says wistfully. 'I'll miss them if you get a new pair. They may only get three or four outings a year, but they've had a place by our front door for fifteen years or more. Just the sight of them as I go in and out each day reminds me that you'll be coming home.'

I reach out and link arms with him, bumping my shoulder gently against his.

'Always Da. This is where you are.'

I take one more circuit of the dining room of The Hydro before returning to Da in the garden. He's standing beside the wall scanning the beach below.

'No luck?'

'No, she's not in there.'

His knuckles are white as he grips the stone.

'Where is she? She's never late. It's more than an hour since she was supposed to be here.'

'I phoned the house again. She's not there. Which way do you think she would come? We could walk back in her direction and hopefully catch her on the way.' I suggest.

Da's right, Mam is almost never late, but he seems to be in much more of a panic than is warranted by a late appearance.

'Are you going to tell me what's the matter? Why are you so concerned?'

Da has pulled a loose thread from the edge of his trousers and is winding it around the index finger of his left hand.

'Your mother has become rather forgetful and absent minded in recent months.'

Da's shoulders drop, and he seems relieved to have finally spoken the words.

'How bad is it?' I ask, horrified at the implications.

'I didn't think it was that significant. She occasionally forgets what something is called, and she doesn't like to cook much anymore, because she finds it hard to get the quantities and the timings right, but most of the time we do ok. I would never have left her alone today if I thought she wouldn't cope. She must have got lost or forgotten where we were going to meet.'

'It's going to be all right Da. We'll find her. I've got my phone, so I'm going to go inside and leave my number with the manager. If she turns up here, they can call me. I think you should walk back home along the beach and once I've left my number, I'll walk back up the road.

Hopefully one of us will find her along the way. If that hasn't happened, and she's not in the house when we get there, then we can get some other people involved and do a methodical search for her.'

'I'm not sure, Isla.' Da seems paralysed by indecision. 'Shouldn't we wait here? Then at least we can be sure we won't miss her.'

I can feel the first twist of new grief running through my core.

'Da, that would have worked in the past if Mam had just got the time wrong, but there's a really good chance she hasn't remembered that she's supposed to be here.'

He nods mournfully.

I give him a quick hug before he descends the steps to the beach, and I head back inside.

As I climb Yerton Brae I pause at every junction, heart fluttering with adrenaline as I peer in all directions, hoping to catch sight of Mam in the navy and white print dress that she was wearing this morning at breakfast.

There is a constant swoosh of traffic as the vehicles speed past me up the main road. The thought of Mam walking along here alone, in a confused state, fills me with dread. The pavements are incredibly narrow. Would she remember to look behind her if she stepped out into the road?

As I reach Overton Drive my heart skips a beat. Up ahead, by the war memorial, I'm sure I can see blue and white. I break into a run, even though there's a significant incline and I'm not very fit.

There, sitting on a bench, looking surprisingly serene, is Mam. I cross the road and lean on the railing so that I can talk to her.

'Hi Mam.'

'Isla, when did you get here?' she asks innocently. 'You should have told us you were on your way. We would have come to meet you at the station.'

'I arrived last night.'

This is bad. She'd even forgotten that I'm here.

'Oh, I'm so sorry that I wasn't awake to greet you.' Mam twists and raises her arms, despite the railings between us. 'Come in here and give me a hug.'

I do as she suggests. There is nothing to be gained from pointing out that we did in fact spend last night together and a further few hours this morning.

'I told Da we'd meet him back at the house. Are you ready?' I ask as I enter the enclosed paved area.

Mam seems unconcerned by my sudden appearance, or the news that I have been speaking to Da, and willingly stands to embrace me. Linking arms with her, for my own sake more than hers, we begin a slow and steady trek back home.

Unfortunately, I find that the depth of my relief is giving me the shakes, so I pull my arm from Mam's before she notices. I'm going to have to talk to Da about getting a mobile of his own. It's ridiculous that I have no way to get hold of him to let him know that I've found her. He must still be frantic.

James - 2016

James stares at the giant puddle covering the floor of the kitchen. The door of the freezer is wide open and obviously has been all night. The increasingly familiar lump is blocking his throat once again and his nails are biting deep into the palms of his hands.

These costly mistakes are happening more and more frequently.

He can feel his breath becoming ragged as his desperation level rises.

Last month Tilly turned on the taps to run a bath and then went out leaving the plug in. He'd returned home to find the bath overflowing and water running all the way down the hall. They'd got off lightly, only having to replace the hall carpet and the lino in the bathroom.

Now, only a few weeks later, the freezer is going to need completely restocking. With everything defrosted all at once, there's no way they're going to be able eat all these ready meals before they go off.

James's despair is making him lightheaded. This wasted food is supposed to last them the next three weeks. It's not like he can magic up another pension payment to cover replacements. If only they'd not done that huge supermarket shop two days ago.

The tears start to cloud his eyes. It's too much!

He knows that he ought to take off his slippers and start cleaning up, but he can't face it. Instead, he retreats to the front room. These early mornings are his only time away from the unpredictable onslaught that has become his life once Tilly wakes.

If he's lucky she may sleep for several hours yet. He glances at his watch. Even though it's only 6am, the one-hour time difference with Germany means that Isla will be up and getting ready for work. He needs to hear her voice.

He picks up the phone.

'Hello there,' he says as she answers, before she has even had a chance to speak.

'Da! What's the matter? You sound exhausted.'

'Your mother was up half the night.'

He can feel the compassion in the silence before she asks.

'What was it this time?'

'She became fixated on looking for you. Well, you know, the teenage you. I couldn't get her to leave your old bedroom for more than a few minutes at a time. She was adamant that you were out at the cinema with friends and due home at any moment. She kept going in there to check if you'd got back.'

'Oh Da!'

'I'm so cross that we didn't come downstairs to make a drink as we usually do when she's restless, because I could have avoided the latest disaster.'

'Oh god, what's she done?'

'At some point last night, before we went to bed, she opened the freezer door. I don't know how I didn't notice. It's completely defrosted. There's water all over the floor.'

'Da these things are happening more and more often. It sounds like Mam really needs watching all the time.'

James feels the muscles across his shoulders clamp at Isla's implication that he's not taking enough care of her mother.

'I have to leave her sometimes Isla. It's not often, but there are times, like taking the car for its service the other morning. She can't walk back anymore. It's too far.'

'I really think you need some help,' Isla persists. 'The damage that would have been done last month had you not come home when you did doesn't bear thinking about. The whole ceiling could have collapsed under the weight of the water.'

James is surprised to find that this time he agrees, so he lets Isla continue without his usual protest.

'Could you find someone to come in, just for a couple of hours a day? It would give you a break, and also create set times when you can make appointments, or go and play golf, anything just for you.'

'I have to admit that does sound nice.' He confesses. 'A chance to meet some other people, and have an occasional conversation that doesn't go around in circles!'

'Da, will you let me pay? It's the least I can do, given that I can't help out in person.'

James hesitates. He hates the idea of Isla paying for things. It makes their relationship feel backwards. He's the parent. He should be the provider for his family.

'Come on Da. There have to be some advantages to having a *fancy pants business executive* for a daughter.'

James smiles. He only used that phrase about her once, years ago, but she is never going to let him forget it.

'It'll make me feel better for not being there.' She urges.

'It would need to be someone your mother trusts.'

'Thank you!'

James can hear the relief in Isla's voice at his decision, and he must admit, it matches his own feeling inside.

Isla - 2017

The glass atrium of the foyer echoes with the brusque clacks emitted by my high-heeled shoes striking the hard floor. As I wait for the lift, to take me the eight stories to my office, I'm thankful for the natural coolness of the huge space. My navy-blue suit jacket and pencil skirt are smart but too warm for the time of year.

Despite the air-conditioning in my car, the summer heat has caused me to break out in a sweat just crossing the car park, so I'm desperately hoping that the rather erratic cooling system on our floor is operating as powerfully as it was yesterday when I chose this outfit.

As I exit the lift, I notice an unfamiliar face at our reception desk. I nod and try to smile in her direction, but I haven't got time to stop. I will say hello properly this afternoon once this is all over.

I hurry down the corridor into my office and close the door.

I feel ever so slightly sick, which is not uncommon for me before a major test of my ability. I think it started when I was a child, when I would often detect, and then mirror, my mother's anxiety - it's something that she's always struggled with.

Now that her anxiety is combined with dementia, Da is having a real problem creating routines to keep her calm. She took weeks to settle at the care home when she moved there last year.

Da felt so guilty, but the move was essential. He'd reached the point when he simply couldn't cope with her on his own at home.

I must give him a call tonight. It has been nearly three weeks since we last spoke. My turn to feel guilty. I've had so much prep to do for today's meeting, I just haven't had the brain space for what's going on over there.

I might as well be honest, I've not presented the best version of myself in any of my interactions during recent weeks. I've been both preoccupied and impatient with some of the juniors on my team. They lack the experience to grasp the significance of today's meeting.

The directors of our company flew in this morning, to take a detailed look around our site. Any minute now, based on the quality of my pitch, they will decide whether to follow my proposal and take us into an international merger, or sell off our branch of the business and cut their losses. This second possibility would result in a huge number of job cuts for staff here in Dortmund.

So, you could say, that today is the culmination of my whole career. The realisation of my personal vision, to help a company set foot on the global stage. That's if it all goes to plan. If not, I will have failed utterly, and many of my colleagues will be without jobs. No pressure there then.

I've got fifteen minutes before I need to join Peter and the others in the conference room. Business management is my thing, rather than the specifics of micro-systems technology, which is Peter's area of expertise. Between us we make quite a team.

I know that our case has the potential to persuade them, despite the recent downturn in the wider companies' profits. Our side of the business keeps huge potential for growth if we think globally.

However, I'm not going to persuade anyone of anything with my mind flitting about like this. I've got to focus. If I just sit like a sponge in front of the documents for ten more minutes…

Without warning there is a knock on the door and the new receptionist walks straight in.

'Ms MacLeod, I'm sorry to interrupt, but there's an urgent phone call for you.'

Pent up with nervous energy and fizzing at the audacity of this woman's bold interruption at a new place of employment, I explode.

'How urgent can it possibly be?'

'Very, I'm afraid,' she adds hurriedly. 'Your father …'

'He's just going to have to wait until later.' I snap. 'I'm about to go into the most important meeting of my life, and I need these few minutes to prepare.' I wave my hand dismissively towards the door. 'Tell him I'll call him back.'

For Da to interrupt me at work, there has to be some kind of issue with Mam, but he will have to handle it alone for an hour or two. After all, there is nothing I can do from here in the short term, and there is so much riding on this meeting.

'I can't …' the woman says plaintively.

'Why the hell not?' I snap. I can't believe I've been so rude, but my fury's got the better of me.

'He's dead.'

Tilly - 2017

Tilly is waiting. These days it's all she seems to do. This room is not a bad place to wait. There are comfortable chairs, and a bed if she feels sleepy, but there's not much to do. The trouble is, she can't actually remember how she likes to spend the time. The other people here seem to be very busy.

Outside her window someone is mowing the lawn in the sunshine. There is nothing like the smell of freshly cut grass to announce the arrival of summer. The flowerbeds are bursting with colour and there are several lovely benches to sit on, but she can't remember how to get out there. It's better to wait here. When James comes, he can take her. He knows the way.

It's noisy here, not like at home, there is always someone talking, or the sound of a television set. Outside the door to this room the corridor is busier than the main street in the village.

Tilly can hear footsteps now, and another noise that she can't identify. She turns in the hope that it's James at last, but it's a woman. Tilly has seen her somewhere before but doesn't know her name.

'Hi Tilly, are you ready to have your rest now?' The woman asks, picking up Tilly's lunch tray and placing it on her trolley.

'I'm waiting for James.'

'James isn't coming today Tilly.' The woman says with regret.

'But he comes every day.'

'I know he used to, but he can't visit today.'

'Tomorrow then.'

The woman pauses, her hands still resting on the trolley. But she doesn't reply.

Tilly accepts that there is no point in waiting for James any longer and crosses the room to her bed.

'I'll see James tomorrow.'

The woman seems very uncomfortable, but still says nothing, and helps Tilly take off her slippers and lie down.

Tilly is tired she can feel herself nodding off.

Darkness opens … edge of the Loch.
Side by side, … Happiness … James.
James gone. … Inchcailloch island?
Family fun … sunshine … Happiness … James.
Blurring … clearing … burial ground … daffodils. …
Desperation … fear.
Relief. James … home … through the village.
Not the village … the water's edge … Loch Lomond. … Happiness.
Dancing. Portencross … Headstones. Suction. Nausea. No!

The war memorial. Loss, more loss. NO! ... NO! ... NO!
Unexplained tears ... aching belly ... James.
The Glen? ... Here? ... Yes! Look, there.
Why is he not waiting?
Not The Glen. The beach. James! Slow down!
The golf course. ... Obviously. ... THE GOLF COURSE, NO!!!
The memorial. ...The golf course. ... Can't Breathe!
Oh! James, you waited! ... Calm. ... Lean on his shoulder. ... Peace.
Smell of whisky. ... Feeling tipsy ... velvet earlobes ... secrets no one knows.
Favourite garden. Little bridge. Flowering springtime.
Gone. ... Where now? The Glen? ...
No! Yet another graveside.
Not James. He wouldn't leave.
James ... James?
Cornfield. By his side ... Happiness ... James.
Sunlight. ... Bird flight ... Happiness ... James
Playful running ... running ... leaving! ... LEAVING ...
Stop! ... Wait! ... Stay!
Porous. ... Wispy. ... Gone.

Someone is shaking Tilly awake. Tilly has seen her before, but she's talking in a strange way. Tilly can't understand. She won't go away. Tilly pulls the covers up over her head. James is dead. There is no more point to living.

Two

Isla - 2017

Everything around me disappears. Pulled at light-speed into a micro-dot just between my ribs. Breathing is not possible, and all I can hear is the intermittent whooshing sound of my own blood pumping in my ears.

I wave the new receptionist away once more, and this time she does leave, understanding that having delivered her message, she will actually have to ask whoever is on the line to wait.

I try to continue my preparation. As I open the first document, it feels as though I am using my computer via a very long robotic arm from another room. The sponge preparation technique I tried earlier isn't working. I can't absorb anything. My eyes are staring, but my brain is not looking.

Poor Da! What on Earth happened? Despite being over eighty, he was so fit. I look down at my hands. My knuckles have gone white because they are clenched so hard into fists. My toes are doing the same inside my shoes, and my ribs are behaving like the tightest corset ever invented. It's obvious that there are not going to be any tears just yet. At least, so long as nobody is nice to me.

I cross the room and lock the door. With a bit of luck, the receptionist will keep this to herself, at least until our meeting has begun.

Five minutes. I need to get back in the game.

I pause mid-presentation. I can hear murmuring from the end of the table. I glance up. It's not coming from Peter, although he's looking very uncertain, and is attempting to make some kind of silent communication between us with his eyes. I think he must know about Da.

The Company Vice-President seems happy. He's smiling, and his head is bobbing almost imperceptibly. He's hooked. A shot of adrenaline surges through my body. I continue my scan of the room.

To my horror, it's the Company President who's muttering. His finger is running down the table of figures as he probes the document in front of him. Thank goodness I've spent the last three months crunching data. If he wants numbers, he's going to get them. I bring up the slide of our sales figures during the last quarter.

I'm about to launch into an explanation when Peter suddenly stands up. I glare at him, as best I can, without showing it to the others.

'I don't know about all of you,' he says expansively, pushing himself back from the table, 'but I could use some refreshment before we get stuck into this new set of figures. I'll be back in a moment. Isla, could you give me a minute in my office please, there's something that I need to check with you.'

Peter uses his foot to close his office door behind him, then sets a cup of tea down in front of me. Peter never makes tea!

'I put sugar in it,' he says, 'it's supposed to be beneficial for shock.'

I smile my thanks. The tea is weak and black. I'm not sure it's going to have the desired effect.

'Isla, I'm so sorry about your father! Why did you start the meeting without telling me?'

'How did you find out?' I ask, ignoring his question.

'Our new receptionist sent me an email when she got the call. She wasn't sure where to find you as you weren't in your office, and she was unsure what you look like. Unfortunately, I didn't pick up the message until we were in the meeting. Otherwise, I would have postponed the start until we could talk. You must be devastated. I know how much you loved your father.'

The truth of his words and the gentleness of his tone are too much for me and I can feel my first tears start to ooze from my eyes. I run my hand along each cheekbone to sweep them away and reach into my jacket pocket for a tissue.

A moment or two later, I bundle a soggy tissue into the palm of my hand, and reach for the handle of the mug, sitting on the table in front of me.

'Give me five minutes to drink this, and I'll be ok to go back in.' I say, blowing on the tea to cool it quickly.

'Don't be ridiculous' Peter shakes his head at me. 'I'll reschedule the rest of the meeting for next week.'

I'm mortified.

'But they're only in town for two days. That's the whole reason why today is so important. They're going to go with the alternative proposal if we don't finish our argument. Right now, we're on a roll. I'm pretty sure the Vice-President's with us already, but he doesn't get to make the final decision.'

'Isla, they're not monsters. Your father has just died. They'll give us a day or two.'

My mind is whirling with logistical issues, but before I can say anything he continues.

'I can go up to head office if necessary to complete the presentation, as long as you talk me through the final section. Your notes are so comprehensive, it won't be a problem.'

'Peter, that won't be necessary. I can do it. In fact, I insist.'

It's out of the question that anyone but me completes the pitch of this project. I've put my heart and soul into it, for the last two years.

'No Isla. Your place is in Scotland right now.'

'Mam's in a care home, and the dementia means that she won't know whether I visit her this week, or sometime later, after we tie things up here.' I point out with grim honesty.

'That may or may not be true, but there are legal issues that have to be dealt with. My wife faced this situation last year. As your father's only relative considered to have decision-making ability, you will have to sort out his affairs.'

I lift my head in astonishment.

'Me? But I don't know anything about his affairs. I happen to know a little bit about Mam's situation, because we discussed it once he realised that he couldn't cope at home, but with Da it was different. He was private about that sort of stuff.' I shift awkwardly in my chair.

The reality had been, that when it came to Mam's care, Da had only needed me as a sounding board. He had actually made all of the decisions alone. I flounder on.

'We never discussed anything about his affairs. He has always been so sharp, and full of vigour. For goodness' sake, he still climbs the Munros in the Trossachs on a regular basis.'

'Well, his heart obviously wasn't as strong as his body.'

Peter's comment brings me crashing back to reality.

'No, I guess it wasn't.'

My tears fall unexpectedly in a devastating torrent. Peter, uncertain what to do, moves to stand beside me and rests a hand on my shoulder whilst I weep.

As I press my now-drenched tissue to my eyes, he reaches into his breast pocket and passes me a freshly pressed linen handkerchief.

It takes a few minutes, but eventually I pull myself together.

'I had better go and apologise to that new receptionist. I was so rude to her. It wasn't her fault. She was in an impossible position. Can you remind me of her name?'

'Her name's Marta, and yes, you definitely need to apologise. Make it a good one! Having said that, Isla, don't be too hard on yourself, your father has just died.

'True, but I didn't actually know that at the time. I was just pumped up about our meeting.'

I feel guilty. Despite having pulled myself up on personal relationships only this morning, I have failed once again to control myself.

'Isla, you're a fighter. You constantly push yourself to your professional limits, and you push others to theirs also. Usually you do it carefully, which gets the best out of your team. Hence all those promotions, and the huge success of this department in the last two years.'

It's satisfying to hear that Peter thinks I've done well. He's not known for gushing support of his team. However, this glowing report doesn't last long.

'Unfortunately though, when you feel a project is under threat, you can be devastating in your dealings with others, and that certainly happened with Marta today.'

I reach out and place his damp handkerchief on the table between us, as I confess.

'All I could think of was the presentation, and how important my arguments were going to be for the future of this site.'

'I understand, and I'm sure that Marta will too. She's young and inexperienced, and I'm sure she won't burst in on anyone else again. No matter what news she's bringing!'

Marta had been really good about my aggressive outburst. Not only had she accepted my apology, but by the time I was ready to head home, she had also bought me a bunch of flowers, and a condolence card. I must mention her kindness to Peter.

Suddenly, I become aware that I have been driving on autopilot. I have no idea how I got here, and worryingly, as usual, I'm in the fast lane of the ring road. I resolve to concentrate, but within a moment my mind has filled with a memory of Da the last time that I saw him, sitting in front of the fire back home in Scotland, with a glass of whisky in his hand.

He was trying to persuade me that despite the winter weather, we should head out early the following morning for a walk before I left for the airport. If only I had said yes!

My eyes mist over, and in an instant, I can't see the car in front, or the one beside me. I put my foot on the brake and the sound of a horn behind me sends a shot of adrenaline through my body. Shaking my head to clear the tears I do my best to make my way to the slow lane, and the nearest exit. I need to stick to the side streets if I'm to make it home safely tonight.

Isla - 2017

Despite Peter's attempts to convince me otherwise, I have delayed my flight to Scotland, until I am certain that the office can run effectively without me, as I will need to be away for the three or four weeks.

However, I have managed to speak to Mam on the phone twice during my lunch breaks. It's been comforting to hear her voice, even though all she said was 'Hello, who is this?' over and over again.

On the second occasion, I also spoke with the care home manager Elspeth. She says that Mam is repeatedly asking when Da will visit. She hasn't retained the fact that he's dead.

I can't think of anything worse than receiving the news again and again, as if for the first time. I honestly don't know how her subconscious can withstand it, given the depth of their sixty-year connection. Perhaps it's better that she doesn't understand.

Three juniors are approaching me, with tablets in hands and harassed looks on their faces. My phone vibrates in my pocket. I'm tempted to ignore it, but it might be Peter.

I glance at the screen. It's Elspeth from the care home. I had better see what she wants. Although, I'm not sure why it can't wait until I see her on Saturday afternoon. I answer, and simultaneously tuck the phone under my ear, holding it in place with my shoulder, as I reach my hand out for one of the approaching tablets, and nod agreement to the graphs I'm being shown on another.

The flight times for my trip to Glasgow sounded excellent, under three hours in the air, the trouble is there is an overnight layover here in Luton. I have almost fifteen hours before my next flight and there is absolutely nothing to do. Normally I would relish this time as an uninterrupted opportunity to work.

However, on this occasion Peter is insisting that if there is any evidence of me online, via the secure system at work, he will force me to stay out of the office for the same amount of time when I return. He knows me too well.

Right now, he wants me to focus on my family, and leave work to look after itself. The trouble is that I don't want to. All I want is mind-numbing distraction.

The word family doesn't mean the same thing to me that it does to other people. Since I was a tiny child, it has just been me, and my parents. Now, given Mam's health situation, thoughts of family just bring me closer and closer to the uncomfortable truth. That before long, I will be completely alone.

Tilly - 2017

Tilly looks more closely at her visitor. She has lovely friendly eyes, and she wants to know about Isla and James. Where are they? They're late. They're going to miss tea with this nice woman. They must be at the beach again. It's always so hard to get them to leave.

This woman's new to the area. Perhaps she would like some recommendations of places to visit. The end of the beach by the golf course is always good. That's probably where Isla and James are now.

If she has a car, she might like to go a little further, the tracks into the hills around Arrochar are easy to explore without getting lost. Isla loves looking for bugs in the forest almost as much as she likes rock pooling.

Portencross … that's the best. Such special memories from when James was working out of the harbour there. Dancing on the grass beside the castle … or was that on the beach in front of the house with the huge turrets? No, that was the day James learnt he would become a father. What an incredible moment that was, she had never felt anything like it. To bring such joy to another person… and now, their little girl is about to be eight years old.

Isla doesn't know it yet, but James has booked a cottage on the shore of Loch Lomond, so that they can celebrate on the island.

Tilly's attention is suddenly back in the room. Who is this strange dark-skinned woman? Why is she asking about Isla? Where's James? What is this place? This isn't home.

Help! Someone? Help!

Isla - 2017

As the train travels along the single track towards West Kilbride, I wonder how Mam and I will manage without the buffer of Da's presence between us. Re-establishing our connection always took us time when I visited. Talking through Da would always allow us the space we needed, until we could talk directly to each other.

I've no idea why my life choices were such a problem for her. From my early teenage years, she fought my wish to study languages and spread my wings, and I have resented her irrational attempts to keep me close ever since.

During the first few years when I was studying abroad, and she refused to visit, I thought that she was just making a point. I thought that after a while she would come around. But she never has.

Over time, I thought more about her anxiety, and wondered if her reluctance to travel was a form of agoraphobia.

However, as public spaces don't seem to cause problems near home, that doesn't seem quite right.

It's only in recent years that some of my deepest hurt, anger and confusion has been calmed by the discovery of a condition called hodophobia. I was told about it by someone that I met at a conference. It is an extreme fear of travel.

Whilst I've never discussed this with Mam, it fits completely with her behaviour, and I just wish that I had realised sooner that a fear of transport and travel could be so debilitating. I might well have behaved differently in response.

She missed out on so much of my life, and Da did too, because she wouldn't travel.

He did come over to visit on his own sometimes, for special occasions: my MBA graduation ceremony, the time I was awarded Employee of the Year, and to celebrate my promotion to European Manager.

My eyes fill with tears. I'm so glad that we had those moments, but I wasted so much time being angry with him too. I thought he was spineless, because he didn't come on his own more often, instead choosing to keep the peace with Mam.

In my darkest hours, I thought that it meant that he didn't really love me, but I know in my heart that wasn't true.

I'm sure, that left to himself, he would have come regularly.

It wasn't that he was *under the thumb* with Mam. After all, I've never known Da do something that he didn't believe was right. He was such a principled man. He just didn't like to leave Mam.

Since the dementia, this of course made sense, but he has always been protective of her, unnecessarily so in my opinion. Despite the anxiety, she's a tough woman my Mam. If her mind is made up, there is no changing it.

Da, on the other hand, is a softy. He'd do anything for you. At least …

My thoughts are all in the wrong tense. I just can't believe that he's gone.

I can feel my throat constricting at the thought of my first solo meeting with Mam. Even without our existing troubles, communication is becoming harder and harder because of the dementia. I'm frightened by the reports of her inability to retain the news of Da's death.

Surely, we are not going to be stuck repeating that painful moment together forever.

Mam usually has an afternoon nap, so I take time to drop my bags at the house, before heading down to see her. The only information that I've retained, from that last, brief, telephone conversation with Elspeth, is that Mam has been struggling with making sense of the present. So, I grab some of her favourite photographs to take with me.

I push open the door of Suncrest Care Home, terrified of what I am about to find.

I must confess that I have avoided thinking too much about Mam's dementia, especially with the pressures of work over the last six months. I focused instead on asking about her physical health whenever Da phoned, confident that they had each other, and were content in their rather impenetrable bubble.

Da had kept a miraculous ability to reach her, despite her increasing confusion and the physical separation that occurred when she moved to Suncrest.

How on Earth am I going to fill that giant hole in her life?

There's no one in the reception area. I can see a member of staff in the corridor leading to Mam's room, so I lift the armful of photographs I am carrying to where they can be seen through the glass, and he buzzes me in.

'I've come to see my mother, Tilly MacLeod.' I can't remember this man's name, but we've met before. Luckily, he recognises me, and nods towards her door.

I press my elbow on her door handle, and push with my shoulder to enter her room.

'Hi Mam,' I say brightly, as I head for the table on the far side of the room to deposit the photographs.

Mam says something that I don't quite hear so I turn to give her my full attention.

She is staring hard at me from the edge of the bed where she is sitting.

'What did you say, Mam?'

She speaks again, but I'm no closer to understanding, as I realise this is definitely not English. She's speaking very quietly so I'm not sure, but it sounds like French, although from the odd word it could possibly be Spanish. I don't think it's Italian.

'Have they had you watching subtitled films in the day room?'

I'd hoped this would raise a smile. One thing I've learned from previous visits is that we need to re-bond quickly. However, far from smiling, Mam starts yelling at me with a stream of utterly incomprehensible, and definitely foreign, words.

How ironic! After all the grief that she's given me for studying languages, now she yells at me, and it's not English.

I try once again to distract her with talk of the photographs, but she's up on her feet, and advancing on me waving her stick in the air. I don't want to upset her like this, and I certainly don't want her to risk falling whilst waving that stick, so I throw up my hands and back towards the door, trying to reassure her as I go.

'Ok, ok I'm leaving.'

Tilly - 2017

Tilly turns. There's a strange middle-aged woman in her room. She's looming towards her. She wants something. Tilly can't understand. The woman's not speaking French. She won't go away.

No more strangers. Why isn't James here? He must have gone to collect Isla. Why has he left her in this place? He never leaves. Darling James. Loyal. Supportive. By her side, day-in, day-out.

He's missing. That's right she remembers now he's missing. He hasn't been to visit in days.

Why did he leave her here? There was a reason. She can't remember. Has he had an accident? Is he in the hospital? She needs to go home. James will find her there.

At last, the woman's gone … but where's home? This isn't it. The room is all wrong. And yet. … That's the chair from the church jumble sale. And that's the vase that James gave her at Christmas.

James should be here.

Isla - 2017

As I return to the reception area Elspeth rushes around from behind her desk to greet me, 'Isla, you're here, how wonderful!'

'Elspeth, what the hell's going on?' I ask. I'm so upset I can feel myself shaking.

'I'm sorry. I did try to explain on the phone.'

'You did?' Why can't I remember? 'Unfortunately, I was heading into a meeting when you called. I had three conversations going on at once.'

I feel incredibly guilty that I didn't give her my full attention at the time. Whatever this is, it's obviously important and deserved attention.

Elspeth fidgets with the edge of her sleeve.

'Don't worry. Adjavella will be back soon.'

I really must remember what Peter says about not being so confrontational. I try to moderate my tone, but this is all so confusing.

'Who's Adjavella?' I'm wracking my brains, am I supposed to know that name?

'She's the specialist communicator we organised for Tilly.'

'Why does Mam need a speech therapist? Has she had a stroke? What about this foreign language?'

'Oh, Adjavella's not a speech therapist, Tilly's speaking fine, it's just that she's talking to us in French rather than English, so we need a translator.'

With my thoughts even more jumbled, I barely hear the rest of her sentence.

'Hang on a minute, you mean she's speaking French all the time?'

'Yes, Tilly seems to have forgotten English.'

'But my mother doesn't speak any other languages. She and Da hated school and left as soon as they could. Da was working with his father on the trawler by the time he was fifteen. My parents weren't academic like me. My passion for study was the main source of conflict, between Mam and me. Especially when it took me abroad.'

'Well, they've been chatting away.' Elspeth insists.

'There's no way that's possible!'

Peter's advice forgotten, I'm now almost shouting. This situation is so ridiculous. I dig my nails into my palms in exasperation.

'I've heard a brain injury can cause someone to speak with a foreign accent, but I've never heard of someone acquiring a whole new language.'

The street door opens behind me. Hearing the click I turn to see a woman in the uniform of the care home approaching with a smile. Elspeth speaks first.

'Adjavella, this is Isla MacLeod, Tilly's daughter.'

The woman extends her hand.

'Oh, I'm so pleased to meet you,' she says with a smile.

I shake her offered hand reluctantly. I'm still not convinced that Mam needs specialist care. If I'm too friendly the pair of them will think I'm on-board with this plan. I've learnt from work that you don't show too much warmth during negotiations until the terms are verging on acceptable.

'Hello.' I reply. 'I gather you've been chatting to my mother. Is it really French? Could it be some kind hybrid of English? Something she's picked up from TV?'

'Oh, no, it's wonderful French.' The woman insists. 'She has a beautiful accent, much better than mine, as if she learnt it directly from a French person.'

I am incredulous.

'The main challenge is finding things to talk about, because I don't know her very well. It's wonderful that you're here. I'm hoping you can tell me all about Tilly and what she enjoys.'

I'm still bemused.

'I can try.' I say, hesitant now that I'm finally calming down. 'I did bring some photographs with me. I remembered that Mam's more connected to her early life than to the present. I thought photos from the house could function as a trigger for conversation.'

'That's a lovely idea.' Elspeth gushes in a bid to smooth things between us.

'I've left them in her room.'

I wonder if they will still be in one piece when we get there, or whether Mam will have thrown them across the room in her rage.

'Then why don't we go and see if we can get her talking?' Adjavella offers.

With some trepidation I follow her back through the double doors and down the corridor to Mam's room. I don't honestly see how the three of us chatting is going to work if they are both speaking French. My mind is still reeling. How can this be possible?

Three

Isla - 2017

As care home accommodation goes, this room is quite pleasant. It has a window overlooking the garden, and Da made sure that Mam has some her favourite possessions around her.

Mam is sitting in one of the two armchairs that were originally in the front room back at the house. She is holding one of the framed photos upside-down in her lap.

I'm pleased that she's calmed down. It gives me a chance to take a proper look at her. Her skin seems sallow, and her cheeks are more sunken than I remember. Worst of all, her head appears to be jutting forward directly from her shoulders. This is a far cry from the proud, upright woman I have always known.

Her head, in this new slump, is also tilted to one side, and her eyes are roving, searching for answers. I wonder if she even knows what the questions are.

My eyes fill with tears, and not just at the change in Mam. I know that in recent months this is where she and Da would sit together for hours, either in companionable silence or listening to tunes on the radio. I can conjure up a vision of him right now in the chair next to her. He has described the scene to me so many times.

When Mam first moved here, Da was taking her back to the house for a few hours each day. However, in recent times, she had started to find that confusing rather than enjoyable, so instead Da had taken to spending time with her here in her room.

He would describe it to me in great detail over the phone, and I have to admit at the time, although I was always delighted that he had called, the repetitive nature of the tales he had to tell often meant that I was not fully listening. My mind was always full of work-related issues. It's a stark reminder that I will no longer be able to just enjoy the sound of his voice coming through the handset.

During our last call, he told me that they had been reminiscing about their tenth wedding anniversary. In fact, it's the image from that day that is in Mam's lap. The photo is of the three of us in the beer garden of a pub that we had gone to for lunch. I was so over excited, it had been building all week with every task that I conducted as *Mam's little helper*, bringing to life the secret plans she had to surprise him.

Tilly - 1968

Tilly is sitting on a bench at the war memorial. Although the lists of those lost in the wars bring sad thoughts of those no longer by her side, it is a great vantage point to appreciate the beauty of the area that she calls home.

As her gaze scans the rooftops of Seamill, there are moments when the sand of the beach, rich and red with the earlier rains, becomes visible between the buildings. She lets her eye continue onwards, panning the view across the water to Arran, and is filled once again with the sensation that she knows so well, the odd mixture of joyful anticipation and reflective sadness.

Tomorrow will be her tenth wedding anniversary. James has booked a table for them at the pub, but she is filled with ideas of her own about how to make it special. She wants to recreate something down by the water, so that they can feel their bare feet in the sand as they did on their wedding day.

She has found a little wicker basket, that Simone would have loved, into which she can place James's present, and will spend this afternoon passing on Simone's skill to Isla, as she teaches her to carefully weave the flower stems in and out of the gaps in the lattice.

This is the first year in which Isla has been old enough to enjoy the celebration, and it has given her such pleasure to share the preparations for each little surprise with her daughter. However, it also serves to remind her of all the people from their wedding day, who are now gone from their lives, that Isla will never get to meet. It is deeply challenging to house two such powerful and contradictory emotions simultaneously, and yet this is the story of her life.

Isla - 2017

Adjavella is kneeling in front of Mam. She starts speaking in French. I watch Mam intently. I'm not sure exactly what is being said, but I recognise my name, and a few other words.

Mam shows absolutely no reaction to my name, and I feel icy fronds creep across my heart. She has forgotten me. And yet, the minute she hears that there are photographs of Da her head flicks around to follow Adjavella's arm as it points to where the images are lying on the round table near the window.

I can't bear it, Da is dead and Mam doesn't recognise me. I quietly slip out into the corridor.

Sad and bewildered, I stand leaning my back against the wall and breathe in deeply. It's not her fault. It's the dementia. She hasn't seen me for over six months, a gap that is too long for someone struggling with their memory.

I collect my thoughts. I find an extra chair in the reception area and return with it to Mam's room. She and Adjavella are already sitting at the table, but the photographs are still in a pile in the middle. I place my chair alongside them, smiling at Mam as I sit down.

They have been speaking in French, but Adjavella switches to English.

'Ok, let's take a look at these shall we?'

Mam has her glasses on. She is peering at me suspiciously over the top of them.

'She doesn't know who I am, does she?' I comment bleakly.

'Not today, no. She was excited when we said you were coming. I know it must be very upsetting not to be recognised. Her memories come and go. Let's see if the pictures help.'

I select one of the photographs and hand it to Adjavella.

'What about this one?' I suggest, 'Da in all his gear about to set off on the trawler.'

It's a lovely photo and I know it's one of Mam's favourites.

'He gave up life at sea to become a fishmonger. He wanted to be around whilst I was growing up.'

James - 1964

James is sitting on the harbour wall. The trawler is due to leave in a few minutes. He should be on board already, but he can't take his eyes from his beautiful wife. Perhaps it's his imagination but her belly seems to be growing visibly each day.

He hears her shriek in frustration. She's experimenting with the new box camera he bought her on her birthday. With a child on the way he wants her to be able to record every moment whilst he's out at sea.

James is worried about her self-imposed isolation. Since they married and moved to West Kilbride, she has resisted any suggestion of getting to know the locals. The only consolation is that Tilly usually spends her time with his mother, and for that he is glad.

His parents were sceptical of his decision to marry someone that they didn't know. However, every day they've been able to observe closely how much Tilly loves him and have both taken her under their wing.

Their support has given him the confidence to come to the harbour today. He can't bear the thought of a week's separation. When the baby arrives, he is certain that he won't be able to do it anymore.

He will have to look for another form of employment, but he has no other skills, and West Kilbride is not exactly brimming with opportunities for unemployed young men.

James poses for one final picture before leaping from the wall, calling his farewells as he runs for the boat, knowing full well, that if he were to take Tilly in his arms one last time, he would never leave.

Isla - 2017

The picture is a success and Mam becomes very animated. It's an amazing transformation from the woman sitting in the armchair when we first walked in. Although I am unsure what she is saying, she is pointing at the photograph and gesticulating. The conversation plays out in front of me like a game of tennis, even though I can't follow a word.

    Nevertheless, it is wonderful to watch as Adjavella asks questions and Mam searches animatedly for the answers.

Tilly - 2017

Tilly's eyes fix on the photograph of James. She is immensely relieved that this winter he will remain in West Kilbride, but it has to be acknowledged that he looks marvellous dressed up in his fishing gear ready to go out on the trawler.

Hang on … that's not right … Isla started school several years ago, so James has been a fishmonger a lot longer than a few months. … He planted the orange roses in the garden the year he stopped fishing. … That orange rose hidden in his pocket as he walked up the lane towards the farm was so special. … Roses for love. …

Orange roses and orange berries in the lane. … The berries that overhang the street on the way to the shops - like a cluster of miniature buoys in the harbour. … James on the harbour wall talking to the seagulls.

Seagulls flying over the white castle with the black turrets. … No, … the red castle with grey turrets. …No, … the castle at Portencross doesn't have turrets at all. It does have a flagstaff though, and a cannon, Isla likes to sit on it.

Isla - 2017

Adjavella is trying to confirm something that has been said, when suddenly Mam's head slumps forward onto her chest.

'Oh, my god, is she ok?' I ask, shocked at her collapse.

'Yes, don't worry. She's just fallen asleep. It's exhausting for her trying to make sense of her memories. Especially as she then has to explain them to me. I'm really sorry that this session has been so short.' Adjavella places the photograph on top of the others. 'I think Tilly has probably had enough for the day and needs her sleep.'

She stands and slips silently behind Mam as she moves towards the door, gesturing for me to do the same. Whispering so as not to disturb Tilly, she continues.

'Let's try again with the other photographs tomorrow. It was a great idea to bring them.'

Isla - 2017

As I approach the house, I'm struck by how beautiful the climbing rose looks in the sunlight. It has grown so much that its upper branches are now curling around the bedroom window above the front door.

Roses are Mam's favourites. There are several in the back garden as well as this one. She seems to be attracted to them like a magnet - she would always stop and admire them whenever we passed some on the street. Even my birthday cards always had a rose somewhere in the picture, until the last few when Da started buying them for her.

The house is cold despite it being July. I'm so glad Da didn't die alone here in the house. It could have been ages until somebody found him. Instead, he was on the golf course with his friends when he collapsed. From what I've been told, they summoned the first aiders and an ambulance very quickly. However, he had suffered a cardiac arrest and despite all their efforts, he never regained consciousness.

I slowly pull my key out of the door and close it gently behind me. My suitcase is still in the hall where I left it two hours ago. I take hold of the handle and heft it up the stairs in front of me. I can't for the life of me think what's in it to make it so heavy. Perhaps I'm just weak from lack of sleep.

Out of habit, I take my old room on the right at the top of the stairs. Apart from a few of my childhood books, the room bears little evidence that I've ever lived here. I left at seventeen for university, and then at twenty-one I headed overseas for my first job. Apart from the odd week here and there, I haven't been back for any length of time.

A wave of regret passes over me. I could have had so much more time with both my parents if only I had been a little less focused on my career, and a little more forgiving of Mam's reluctance to travel.

The truth is, that throughout my twenties, there had been an escalating battle of wills. I became more and more resolute that I wouldn't go home until Mam had been to visit me. Eventually, of course I realised that she wasn't coming, and that if I wanted to see her, I would have to give in and travel back to Scotland.

Tilly - 1987

Tilly is lying in bed staring at the ceiling. Unusually, James is still asleep beside her, despite the bright early morning sunlight that is pouring through the thin curtains of their bedroom. He is normally the one to wake with the dawn.

She reaches for her watch. It's not even 5am. She has barely slept. Isla is due back today. Her first visit for over two years. The estrangement has been agony, but Tilly is equally anxious at the thought of their reunion.

The two of them have been too similar in their willingness to let fear control their actions. A lifetime with Isla has taught her that her daughter digs in her heals when she fears that others are trying to control her, and she knows that her refusal to visit Isla will have seemed like a bid for control as she has refused to offer an alternative explanation.

Her inability to sleep these last two nights has been the result of her own fear that Isla will pursue her quest for answers. James is sworn to secrecy, but Tilly knows that he is deeply unhappy about it, and when they are all together, she lives with the constant fear that he will crack under the drilling of their daughter's laser sharp cross-examination.

Isla - 2017

I start to unpack. I hang my business suits in my childhood wardrobe next to some old clothes of Mam's. My suits seem so out of place here, and yet at home I rarely wear anything else. I'm wearing my one pair of jeans, and the trainers that I bought, when I thought that I was going to take up running, but it turned out that I didn't have time.

I'll have to see if there are any local shops where I can buy myself a more appropriate item or two tomorrow.

Apart from my washbag, the rest of my suitcase is empty and yet it's still very heavy. Curious, I unzip the inner lining and uncover a stack of paperwork between the lining and the metal frame of the wheeling mechanism.

I smile. Peter may have stopped me from going online, but I am going to be able to work after all. I tucked these documents in here two weeks ago for a flight from Italy. I was transporting olive oil in the main compartment, so I wanted them to be protected if one of the bottles broke. I completely forgot. I spent ages looking for these documents, before eventually printing them off again.

Now, thanks to my failing memory – a shadowy concern given Mam's situation – I won't be too far behind the pace when I get back.

As Mam's not up to another visit today, I decide to head to the golf course. I want to see where Da died.

To avoid the traffic, I follow my wiggly childhood route to Summerlea Road. I think of all the times that I walked along the lane here holding Da's hand and looking out for rabbits hopping across the field.

Da told me a few weeks ago that they're planning to build hundreds of new homes on the land in this area. The people losing their sea views aren't going to be happy. I wonder if they'll receive any compensation.

I take the footpath that overlooks the garden, stopping to admire the stream and its narrow wooden footbridge. Beyond this point the water flows out across the golf course. It has been diverted into a well-maintained and neatly banked channel, in order to ensure that it reaches the sea without too much interruption to play.

The sight of the golf course causes my lower lip to shake, and my vision to blur. A group of men in the midst of play are heading my way, so I retreat swiftly to the shelter of the trees to collect myself. I wait until they've moved on, and then follow the stream straight down to the sea. I need more time before tracing Da's last steps.

The red-tinted sand is so familiar, I can't resist taking off my trainers and socks and feeling its roughness as it works its way up between my toes and polishes the soles of my feet. Cheaper than any pedicure.

I make a beeline for my favourite slab of rock that, true to form, has a little rockpool at its most seaward point. I dip my feet in and make wet footprints on the slab. Then I do the same with my hands. Family traditions are important, even, or perhaps especially, when you are the only one left that knows about them.

I had forgotten the extent to which this view can fill me with calm. The long row of hills on Arran, which stretch into the distance across the water, offer this section of coastline, protection from the power of the open ocean, and somehow, I feel protected too.

Despite giving up life on the trawlers more than fifty years ago, Da rarely went a day without communing with the sea. He was an early riser and had usually been down to the beach and returned home, long before I was out of bed, or had had my breakfast, even on school mornings.

But it was the days when he broke routine that I remember the most. Those were the days we came to the beach together after school, sometimes in the dark with a torch, sometimes early enough to catch the sunset, but always to breathe in the calmness of the ozone in the air, and to let the sound of the waves play in our ears.

I sit now and watch the gentle rise and fall of the water. I've lived in large cities all my adult life, yet it is this landscape that is part of my identity. I feel it resonate within me. I've missed it whilst I've been away.

James - 1970

James is kneeling uncomfortably on a barnacle-covered ledge, up to his armpit in a rock pool. He is using a flimsy child's fishing net to chase a small crab that his daughter has spotted.

With her arms around his neck, Isla is draped across James' back, peering over his shoulder. Occasionally she lets go with one arm to point excitedly at her escaping prey.

These times together are so precious. The rapid processing of his daughter's mind fascinates James. The speed with which she connects events and interprets new information is quite astonishing.

This is not just the warm glow felt by every proud father. He recognises in his daughter an intelligence that cries out to be fed. She may only be six years old, but it is clear to anyone that meets her, that she will not be content with a quiet life here in West Kilbride.

With every passing year, it becomes harder to keep his own counsel. Isla is naturally curious, and can spot a diversionary tactic a mile off, whilst Tilly is becoming increasingly twitchy about the threat this brings to the calm stable life that they have created here.

The stability of his wife's fragile mental health is essential for the on-going success of their family life here in West Kilbride. Although he is not technically lying to his daughter and the wider community, he is most definitely withholding the truth. That Tilly's peace of mind is secured by his own complicity causes a deep conflict between James's heart and his moral code.

Isla - 2017

I cast my eye along the waterline towards the Hydro. Today is a busy day at the other end of the beach. The children are on holiday, and sandcastles and trenches have changed the landscape of the shore, but only until the next high tide. Then all will be gone, just like my family.

The sweeping tide of fate has rolled in and taken my father, and all of my mother, save for her physical body. I didn't see it coming. Not for one minute did I think that Da would be gone. If you had asked me, I would have guessed that he had at least another ten years.

I feel cheated. There was so much that I wanted to do with him. I had even started to think about coming back here for regular long weekends in the years to come, so that he wouldn't be lonely now that Mam is no longer real company.

He would have laughed, and not believed me if I had mentioned it to him, as I have been such an infrequent visitor over the last thirty years. But it's true. The idea has been in the back of my mind for several months because I could feel that times were changing.

Creating the blueprint for an international merger has been my ultimate career goal. I needed to prove that I could do it. Assuming that all goes as expected in the coming weeks, much of the challenge of my current job will be gone, and I have absolutely no idea what I'm going to do next.

I've never been one for repeating myself. After all, where would all the challenge or excitement be? How ironic that I reach this decision point in my life a few years too late.

Just like tourists on the beach, stranded by a sudden rise in water level, I find myself unexpectedly cut off and alone on an emotional island.

When I was young, it was so important to me that I achieve success and recognition through my career. It sounds big-headed, but the truth is that I was much brighter than the other children in my class at primary school. As a result, I became bored with their interests, and therefore chose to play alone, something that I was used to doing at home when I didn't seek out my father.

As a teenager I sought the company of students a few years above me, always on a quest to learn, and to stretch myself. I regularly prioritised opportunities for advancement over chances to socialise, and this remained true when I moved abroad.

It was ten years before I could really say that I had a circle of friends in Hamburg, and then a promotion took me to Berlin, and I had to start again.

Had I wanted children, this would have been the time to find a partner, but I wanted success in my own right, and so I put my head down and worked long into the nights.

It paid off, and the 'Employee of the Year' award saw me move yet again, this time to Dortmund, with the European Manager position giving focus to my life just two years ago.

I live for what I do, and I love it. There is nothing like assessing the talent within a company, taking the whole business apart, restructuring it, and making it many times more successful than anyone else ever thought it could be, purely because the employees are now doing what they do best, and working to their full capacity.

However, on reflection, the price I've paid is a heavy one. I am alone.

I lost touch with the Hamburg circle because I never went back for visits, and despite having lived in the same apartment block in Dortmund for two years, until last week, I'd not even met my next-door neighbour.

If I'm totally honest, the contact with my neighbour would never have happened if Da hadn't died. I only introduced myself as a preamble to asking if she would keep an eye on my cherished apartment.

Over the years, I have created a space that is an oasis of calm tranquillity. A stark contrast to the stress of the office. Unfortunately, because I have used so many plants to generate the atmosphere that I want, there is no way that it can survive my absence for this long without someone to top up the reservoirs in the automatic watering system.

I wonder if there are many *tiny islands* like me in the world population, cut off by the tide of life.

Four

Isla - 2017

Once again, I'm in Mam's room, photographs at the ready. As Adjavella explains why we're here and encourages Mam to make her way to the table, I reflect on the discovery of the documents in my suitcase last night.

How did I not remember that I had put them under the lining? To forget temporarily is one thing, but to forget completely, that can't be good. I wonder what age Mam was, when she first started forgetting things. I'm sure she wasn't as young as I am.

I've been very preoccupied with work. I really hope that's all that it is. Maybe I should find the courage to speak to Elspeth. She's a professional after all.

Oh, I wish Da were here! We could have gone for a walk, and when we were right out on the end of the headland, where only the wind could hear, I could have confessed what happened, and asked when he first noticed that Mam had a problem.

I can't ask Mam. Even if she still had the necessary self-awareness, she no longer has a single word of English. However, I have high hopes that Adjavella will have more tales to translate in a moment.

Once Mam is settled Adjavella selects a beautiful picture from my parents thirtieth wedding anniversary trip to Loch Lomond.

Tilly - 2017

Tilly stares at the item in her hand.

Thoughts rush. Ideas blur. ... Her head feels woolly. ...She's looking, but she can't see. ... Her eyes aren't working ... She shakes her head in the hope that they will focus and do their job, and her thoughts will come back together.

She twists the thing in her hand, unsure what to do with it. ... The people are talking, but the sounds don't make sense. ... She can feel the panic rising.

This is happening a lot lately. Is it lately, ... or has it been a long time? Where's James? Her chest feels tight.

Isla - 2017

Adjavella gently removes the photograph from Mam's hand.

'I'm sorry Isla, Tilly doesn't seem to be connecting to this one. Perhaps she doesn't recognise James at that age.'

'What about this one?' I say reaching desperately for another image. 'Da's much younger here, it might even have been taken before the one we showed her yesterday.'

Tilly - 2017

Tilly is trying to explain one of her favourite activities to these women. She loves to watch her husband walking ahead of her down a track, or away into the distance along the shoreline.

Okay, it's true, she likes to watch the sway of his gait, but it's more than that, James is the kindest man that she has ever met, and he tells everyone that he is happiest when he is with her, but she knows his secret. He is most happy when he is at one with nature. It is this joy that she watches, as he walks ahead of her down a track.

Her body, and her emotions, understand this concept. Yet today, she cannot find the words to express it. The ideas are all there, but they are layering up and they can't get out.

Every separate memory of James walking a short way ahead of her, is presenting itself with equal determination, screaming to be the story told today.

As one memory reaches the surface of consciousness, so another comes crowding in. A logjam of ideas, banging and crashing against each other, and at the same time, softening and merging into one another.

Some are like butter and sugar creamed together, until eventually neither one exists anymore. Others are stretched wide like spiders' webs, waiting to tangle threads around each other. Partial images make it to the surface, only to fall back into the soup and disappear beyond rescue.

Isla - 2017

Unfortunately, despite these lovely pictures, Mam shows almost no response today. In the end we give up. As we walk down the corridor to the reception area Adjavella says,

'Try not to be too sad. Some days Tilly is talkative, but on other days she can be quite moody, or just silent like today.'

I believe her when she says that Mam's days vary, but despite this, I have seen that Adjavella receives the odd smile from Mam. Yet so far, there has been nothing for me, her daughter.

Isla - 2017

This waiting-room magazine is at least two years old. I wish I'd brought some of my work files with me, but I came here on impulse as a plan B when this morning's visit to Mam didn't go so well.

I really have no idea where to start with making a connection to Mam, so I've come to speak to Da's GP in the hope of finding out what happened. Although I don't have an appointment, he has promised to fit me in during his lunch break, so it shouldn't be long now.

The doctor's tone of voice is very matter of fact.

'Silent Myocardial Infarction or SMI is a type of heart attack that has few symptoms but can leave scarring in the heart.'

It is just the kind of tone that I use at work, to keep discussions away from the emotional issues related to a project, when they are likely to cloud people's judgments of the facts. However, the tone is hard to listen to when he's talking about my Da.

'Further problems often develop if a cardiac event goes unnoticed. It appears your father must have had a few of these episodes.' He nods his head in quiet agreement with himself.

'You mentioned that there could have been multiple symptoms. What might they have been?'

I wish I'd known what to look out for.

'Rather than the pain that is more commonly associated with heart attack, there can be what patients describe as discomfort in the centre of the chest, but this is often mistaken for gastric reflux.'

'There was a bottle of Gaviscon beside the bathroom sink when I arrived. It was almost empty.'

'Patients often complain of aches in the neck, back or arm ...'

I interrupt.

'Da was complaining to me on the phone recently about how he must be doing something wrong with his golf swing as he was experiencing aches in all three. He even talked about taking a lesson or two to put it right.'

'If only he had told us. I would have put two and two together.'

I wonder who the *us* is but continue with my original train of thought.

'So is a string of SMIs always fatal?' I ask.

Now it's my turn to try and stick to the facts. I can feel myself getting unhelpfully emotional.

'No, but in your father's case each episode inflicted a little more damage, finally causing a sudden and catastrophic cardiac arrest. That bit was very quick.'

I'm pleased to hear this. Overall, it seems that Da was spared a lot of pain and fear. It doesn't make his sudden loss any easier to comprehend, but it is a little easier to bear.

'I've not had anyone close to me die before. Can you tell me what I have to do about registering his death, or anything else I should be doing?'

'Oh, you don't need to worry about any of that, you aren't one of James' executors.'

I flinch at the insensitivity and wonder how he knows.

'I'm not?'

'James discussed his options with me over a round of golf last year. Your mother had just moved into Suncrest, and he was updating all his legal documents. I have you down as next of kin, but James' friend Andrew has already sorted those things as his executor. James asked him to take on the role because you live abroad.'

'So, Andrew is managing everything?'

'I believe so yes, with the help of James' solicitor.'

'Well thank you very much, you've been most helpful.' I stand and stretch out my hand.

If I'm not an executor, I should be back in Dortmund ensuring that the deal goes through. I want to be here for the funeral, of course, and for Mam, especially now that I discover she has this crazy French thing going on. But surely only a few days would have been enough.

Back at the house I flick through the address book on the table beside the telephone. Despite my best efforts, I never did succeed in persuading Da to buy a mobile. There he is. Andrew Hawcroft - lifetime friend of my father, usurper of my daughterly role. This may have been a very logical, practical decision on my father's part, especially given the way that I have behaved in recent years, but it really hurts. I dial the number.

'Hello?' His voice comes down the line enquiring and friendly.

'Good evening, Andrew. It's Isla MacLeod.' I reply adding a little distance with formality.

'Isla my dear, I'm so glad that you called. I'm terribly sorry about your father. Are you in the UK?'

'Yes, I'm at the house.'

'I'll come over, give me just a moment.'

'No, no, it's fine honestly Andrew, but perhaps we can meet up tomorrow and discuss a few things. I gather I'm not actually an executor.'

'That's true, but only because James thought that it would be too complicated with you living in Dortmund. It wasn't to exclude you.'

He must have been able to hear the accusation in my voice.

'I guess I just want to be part of it. To say goodbye.'

'Well, let's meet. We can work out what's to be done, and who will do what. We can go to the lawyer together, but other things won't take two of us. You can choose the things you feel are important for you to do, and I'll pick up the rest. How does that sound?'

'Perfect.' I say in a very small voice. I've been so childish, and he really is a lovely man. I regret that I've been so cross with him.

Sitting up in bed, surrounded by my illicit paperwork, I think of all the other evenings, during the 1970s and 80s, when I had sat in the same position.

Places to do my homework had been hard to find. Mam had been happy for me to share the kitchen table, but there was always a risk of getting flour and grease marks on my work.

The writing desk in the living room was an obvious alternative, but Da was usually in there listening to the radio or watching television. So, I would come up to my room, and climb under the covers to stay warm. In those days there had been no central heating.

My parents stuck to that same after-work routine - Mam in the kitchen with the stove and Da in the living room by the fire - for the best part of forty years. Later in the evening, having done the washing up, she would join him for an hour or so, before they both retired to bed, in preparation for their early start the following day.

There had been little to break this rhythm, and it was obviously something that gave them both great comfort and security, but the mere thought of such a life makes me feel desperately claustrophobic.

Isla - 2017

It has been a few days, and I push open the door of the care home with some trepidation. I have no excuse, I should have been here yesterday and the day before, but sleeping in their house without my parents has been way harder than I anticipated. I have been having trouble getting my head around the idea of a future without either of them to talk to, or to share things with.

Da's death is challenging, but at least I can see that there will be a process to my grief. What is happening here, with Mam, has me feeling both scared, and out of control. Neither of which I am comfortable with. I have no idea what I will find today.

'Morning Isla!' Elspeth is sickeningly bright and sunny this morning.

'Morning.' I can't match her joyful tones.

'Are you ok? We were worried about you.'

'I suppose I knew that Mam was safe here with you,' I admit, 'but I should have called.'

'Her safety is certainly our priority.' Elspeth bobs her head, making a show of tidying the papers on her desk.

Oh dear, I have obviously deeply upset her.

'How is she?' I ask hoping to make amends.

'She's talking about family in Brittany.'

French family? This makes no sense unless they're very distant cousins. Mam has always discouraged discussion of her family, other than days out to Renfrewshire to look at the Tilde graves. Her response was always *it's just me now.* In fact, the use of those exact words, reiterated repeatedly, should perhaps have caught my attention for their repetitive nature. It's possible that the truth might have been expressed with more variation.

'I wish Da were here. He must have known something about French relatives surely?'

If they do exist, wouldn't he have said something about them somewhere along the line? Wouldn't he and I have taken a trip to France to meet them, even if Mam refused to travel?

The door from Mam's corridor opens.

'Adjavella, how are you?' I ask.

She looks tired. It occurs to me that there is no one else who speaks French to share Mam's care. She must be doing plenty of overtime.

'I'm well, but I need to warn you, Tilly is having an acute episode with her vascular dementia. I've tried with the photographs several times. She's lost all memory of your father. Although she's fixated on a goat in the background of one of the photographs.'

The first few times Mam had one of these acute episodes Da was terrified. Her capabilities would crash dramatically. In a matter of moments, she had no idea what the telephone was, or how to put the milk back in the fridge. He had called me in a panic on both occasions. We had both thought that would be it. That we had lost her to her confusion.

However, we soon learnt that unlike with the Alzheimer's - which she also has - where the decline is steady and in a single direction, she can recover from the vascular episodes, at least to some degree.

So, she was soon using the telephone again, and at least for some more months could be trusted to put the milk back after using it. Although she was not so consistent in her ability to close the fridge door afterwards.

I pull my attention back to Adjavella.

'If she's got even a flicker of connection, we've got to try it.'

Mam is lying on her bed. She doesn't look up as we enter the room, and I'm not even sure if she has registered that we're here.

'Hi Mam!' I say placing a gentle hand on her arm in the way that she used to do for me when I was a small child, ill in bed. I remember finding it so comforting.

But she doesn't respond, so Adjavella tries French.

'Bonjour Tilly!'

'Je m'appelle Tilde!' Mam replies crossly.

At least she's responding. I know enough French to know that she was correcting Adjavella about her use of the name Tilly.

'Your mother wants to be called Tilde.' Adjavella says with a sigh. 'She doesn't recognise Tilly as her name. I think that ties in with not remembering your father. She mentioned that he was the one who first called her Tilly.'

I can't help the tears from forming. It's just so unfair.

I fetch a couple of chairs from beside the table so that we can sit near the bed, and Adjavella tries again with a photograph.

This time it works, and Mam becomes quite animated as she shares her memories, but Adjavella is looking more and more confused. After ten minutes or so it becomes obvious, even to me, that whatever Mam is saying, is nonsense. A string of gibberish that is totally incomprehensible.

On my first day back, overcome by melancholy, wallowing in self-pity, I reflected on myself as an isolated human island, formed by the tides of fate.

Poor Mam is experiencing isolation on another level altogether. She is cut off, not only from an understanding of her immediate surroundings, but also from the connections that she has made over the years to everyone that she knows and loves. Worst of all, she is disconnected from herself, her passions, her opinions, and everything that went into making her who she was.

I don't want her to see me cry, so I slip quietly from the room. Sadly, there is absolutely no harm in my doing this, as Mam wasn't really aware that I was there anyway.

Tilde - 2017

Tilde looks at the photograph. … She's not going to worry about these two strange women. … She can't remember who they are, although one of them is here every day. She's nice. She smiles a lot.

Who's the other one? Perhaps she's a friend of Olivier's. … She hopes the woman isn't his girlfriend. That would really stop him noticing her. … But the woman is old. He wouldn't be interested. … Why on Earth had she thought he would be? … Tilde knows that Olivier is a few years older than her, but at seventeen that's old enough to make his own decisions. They could get married if he liked … That could be the answer to everything. … Where is he? … Is this the marriage office? … These aren't working people …

The smiley woman is asking about the photograph. … Tilde can't see it very well, but that looks like the farm. … there, in the corner, surely that's the goat. He is always escaping. …
Tilde can feel her heart expanding.
Warmth, … in the barn, … in the hayloft, … or next to the goats.
Making cider and wine for the adults, … collecting eggs and peeling potatoes. …Home.
Chopping logs for the fire, … cleaning tack for the horses. … Grind stones to sharpen all the blades. … Home.
Blue skies, … thick mud, … woebegone sheep. … Home.

Isla - 2017

A short while later Adjavella enters the reception area to find me sitting on an upright chair drinking a cup of disgusting coffee from a dispensing machine.

'Isla, are you ok?'

'No,' I shake my head ruefully, 'I don't know what's going on. That wasn't even French, was it?'

'I agree it wasn't. I could guess part of what she was saying. There was a lot of talk about animals. Did your grandparents live on a farm?'

'I never met Mam's parents, they died before I was born, but I'm pretty sure they were from the coast too. She talked about watching the weather approaching across the sea from her bedroom window as a teenager.'

'I think Tilly was talking about being in love with a young farm worker. I guess that's not your father, but I can't be sure, I've not heard those particular words before. I think she might be speaking a regional dialect.'

A dialect, oh thank God, not complete nonsense yet.

'It's the same sort of mix of familiar and unfamiliar sounds that I hear when people speak patois.'

'How could she possibly have learnt that?'

This whole situation is becoming more and more bizarre by the minute.

'To be as fluent as she is, she has to be a native speaker.'

I can feel the blood draining from my brain. In a desperate bid to stop the world from spinning, I take a deep breath, rest my elbows on my knees, and clasp my head in my hands.

'I'm sorry, I know that makes no sense to you.'

Adjavella places a comforting hand on my shoulder.

Isla - 2017

I push open the door to Mam's corridor. Today is Adjavella's day off and I'm dreading it. How am I going to communicate with Mam, especially now that she is not even using French consistently?

Elspeth was so pleased that I would be here today. I think the staff members are as uncertain of being alone with Mam as I am. Elspeth asked me to come in at lunchtime to help keep everything calm.

To be honest, I'm concerned that I will have the opposite effect on Mam, as she really doesn't remember who I am, but if it makes the staff feel better, I should be here.

Elspeth is sitting with Mam at the table, a plate of vegetable hash between them, but Elspeth is having trouble persuading Mam to eat it.

As I cross the room to say hello, Elspeth lifts a forkful encouragingly towards Mam's mouth. Mam flicks up her arm and pushes it away. The fork spills its contents onto the table.

'Bonjour Tilde,' I say brightly, hoping to distract her.

Mam shoots a glance in my direction but dismisses me as unknown. She may be struggling with her memory but she's not stupid. Mam returns her suspicious look to Elspeth who has indeed refilled the fork. Once again, she is approaching Mam with intent.

This time it seems Mam has had enough. Perhaps because I am here too, she feels ganged up on, but whatever the reason, she reaches her hand out towards the plate, grabs a handful of hash and hurls it towards Elspeth, who ducks as it flies across the room.

'Oh my god, I can't believe she did that!'

'Please don't worry, it's an occupational hazard.' Elspeth says as she bends to clear up the mess.

'No really, I'm so sorry, this behaviour is absolutely not her. Mam has always put politeness above everything. The woman who brought me up would be mortified to think she was behaving this way. When I was a child, she was always telling me to eat what I was given and be thankful for it.'

'Isla, truly it's fine. However, I do need to clear this away. Why don't we give Tilly some space, and you can try again in a few minutes with some ice cream, she usually likes that.'

Back at the house I reflect on Mam's outburst. The hardest thing about this disease is the way that it strips away an individual's personality. My mother has always been a complex person, but she has been utterly consistent in her complexity.

She might hold contradictory opinions depending upon the issues being compared but there has always been an impressive consistency to those beliefs. It made her very hard to argue with, even when there was absolutely no logic in her demonstrably conflicting opinions.

I spent so much time during my teenage years trying to explain the inconsistencies in her standpoints, but it was like trying to turn a cruise ship using a sailing dingy as a tugboat.

It didn't matter how much proof I had on my side, if something was the way that Mam did it, it was likely to be the way that it would always happen. I found this character trait baffling and immensely frustrating.

Yet now that it has gone, I feel betrayed. It feels as if she has gone back on the only thing that I could count on. An unspoken promise, that if I loved her, despite her challenges, she would pledge to be dependable and predictable in exchange.

Five

Isla – 2017

It has been an emotional fortnight, but after many hours perusing websites and several discussions over gin and tonics in the evenings, Andrew and I sorted out all of Da's affairs, and chose the brand-new Clyde Coast and Carnock Valley Crematorium for his funeral.

As I enter the chapel, I'm once again taken by the magnificent setting. Behind Da's coffin, spread out in front of me through a wall of glass, is the coast, with the mountains of Arran visible across the water. There are fine white curtains to filter the light on the brightest days, but today they are pulled to one side to expose the full impact of the view. It's perfect for Da. He was always a man of the hills and the sea, nothing else made him happier, except Mam, and possibly me.

It feels wrong that after almost sixty years of marriage Mam isn't here to say goodbye to him, but she has no memory of Da and wouldn't understand what's going on. To be honest I'm glad that I can have this time alone to remember him, without worrying about her needs.

Their wedding anniversary would have been next month. I found a note in Da's diary of a booking he had made at the Seamill Hydro – lunch for three. I guess he was intending to invite me over to celebrate with them, although typically he hadn't got around to it. He never did understand how much notice I need to be sure to make it. I must remember to cancel that booking.

Of course, I'm not alone. Da was a wonderful man. At the shop he had a warm, friendly, outgoing persona that has resulted in a packed chapel today. The locals have come out in force to celebrate the life of their friendly fishmonger, and they are seated in comfort.

There are no hard pews in this new chapel. Instead, rows of broad pine chairs with wicker seats span either side of a wide aisle down which the pallbearers can bring the coffin without obstacle.

There are even TV monitors in the large waiting room transmitting the service. A couple of parents with young children have opted to watch proceedings from there, so that their little ones can have the freedom to run around without disturbing the rest of the mourners. Da would have loved that. He always believed in children being free to express themselves.

Despite Mam's reservations, he had encouraged me to spread my wings. Perhaps it was the sailor in him, but when I told him that I wanted to apply for a sandwich degree working abroad, he had fought to make it happen.

It had come as such a surprise. That was when I finally understood the true depth of his love for me. For he rarely took a stand against Mam, at least not in front of me – who knows how it worked between them in private.

I was extremely grateful when Andrew offered to give the eulogy. Today is not a day for putting on a brave face and suppressing my emotions to speak in public. Today is a day for remembering Da and how much I love him. My love is in the present tense, even though our time together is now in the past.

As Andrew speaks, my tears flow without restraint. My heart is thrown on a rollercoaster of emotion, as he recalls long forgotten memories from the life that he shared with my parents here in North Ayrshire.

Members of the congregation are chuckling. Andrew is an excellent raconteur. I'm so pleased that Da is being remembered with laughter and joy and not just sadness and tears.

He was a complex man. To those close to him, he was thoughtful, warm, generous-spirited and loving. He was friendly and helpful to his neighbours and customers, and yet a bit of an enigma to strangers.

At heart, Da was self-contained. He didn't need others, except Mam. He was often away in his own head, and at those times hard to reach.

However, once a bond was set up it was never broken, as can be seen by the numerous people here today to celebrate their own special forms of connection with the man that was my father.

The funeral elicited more concentrated emotion than I have ever known. Following that with a public wake, where I would be bathed in other people's emotions had seemed impossible, but I had managed.

Now, limp as a ragdoll, I am resting on the low wall outside Suncrest. I haven't been able to bring myself to go in, but I can't go back to the house either.

It's real. Da has gone, and in all important respects Mam has too.

The first day that I came here after Da died, I'd had hope that I could reach her. She was moving around her room on her own, peering intently at different objects, watching people in the garden from her window. Although she had been uncertain, she had been actively trying to make sense of things.

Unfortunately, in the few short weeks since then, there have been marked changes. I've no idea what the future holds for the pair of us.

The main door of the care home opens, and Adjavella comes out. She spots me, so I wave, and she comes over to join me.

'What's the matter Isla? You didn't come in.'

'I just can't face it at the moment.' I confess. 'How do you do it? Spend so much time with someone who's not really there.'

'Well, she is not my mother, and I didn't know her when she was well, so that helps. But also, in Senegal we live as families - the old people, with the children, and everybody in between - it's normal to be around people in failing health. You say that she's not here, and maybe that's true of her mind. But her soul – that's still here. I see the Tilly in her heart. She struggles to connect with us, but she is definitely here.'

I wonder whether this is true. Adjavella certainly believes it.

'Have you been a carer for long?' I ask.

'Not so long. My husband was older than me and he had sickle cell disease, which unfortunately led to a stroke. I spent the last six years of his life taking care of him at home. After he died, I needed purpose and an income. I like to look after people, so this job seemed to be an ideal solution.'

'I'm so glad that you made that choice.'

I reach out and for a moment squeeze the hand that is resting beside me on the wall.

'You make such a difference to Mam's life. She's so calm when you're around. You can see the comfort she receives from you in the way that she looks at you.'

Adjavella looks pleased but a little uncomfortable, and I'm equally surprised at myself for my uncharacteristic openness.

'I see a lot of death,' Adjavella says, filling the awkward silence. 'It has made me realise that we only have one life, and we should make the most of it.'

She has a point. The last few weeks have made me realise this too. Whilst I'm pleased to have had the career success that I sought; I should have balanced it with time for personal relationships.

Our conversation here on the wall is the most open conversation I have ever had with a stranger. Not that Adjavella is a stranger any longer. In fact, to my surprise, she feels like a very dear friend.

Perhaps this change in my behaviour is a response to the depth of kindness Adjavella has shown in her dealings with Mam, and with me. Or maybe, the shock of Da's death has brought my own barriers crashing down. Whatever the cause, I have found myself desperately searching for new connections.

'Talking of living our lives,' I say, risking her disapproval. 'I've got to get back to Dortmund. They need me and you're so much better than I am, at getting through to Mam. I'm worried though about her not eating.'

'Oh, I worked that one out. She was having trouble identifying the foods on her plate. She wasn't prepared to eat something that she didn't recognise.'

Adjavella says this is if it is perfectly reasonable, and I suppose that on one level it is. However, I'm horrified.

'You mean she doesn't know what mashed potato is anymore?'

'It's more that her brain's not interpreting what her eyes see. At least not in the same way as before. It'll be easier for her if we keep different foods separate on the plate. I might try changing the colour of the plate itself, that can help too. Whatever happens, I'm definitely going to stop ordering foods like that hash!'

'I still can't believe she threw it at Elspeth.' I say, involuntarily running my fingers through my hair, as if it were matted with mashed potato.

Adjavella stirs, as if to leave, so I quickly reach into my pocket.

'Adjavella, I've got a gift for Mam. Would you be able to keep an eye on it for me? I had a locket made for her. A pinch of Da's ashes were added to the metal by the jeweller. She won't remember that it's from me, or even realise that it belongs to her. But hopefully she will find it beautiful and enjoy wearing it.'

'Oh, what a lovely idea.'

I hold the locket in the palm of my hand so that Adjavella can see.

'There's a photograph of me as a child inside it, from the times when we were so happy and easy in each other's company. The clasp is hard to open.' I demonstrate the mechanism. 'I doubt if she'll even try. There's not much chance she'll know who I am if she sees it, but I will know that the photograph is in there. It will give me comfort knowing that it's in the room with her. A little bit of Da, and a memory of me. The three of us together.

My final task before leaving is to scatter of the rest of Da's ashes. He needs the freedom of the sea, so I head to the shore below the golf course where he died. I feel like his spirit is here already. I stand with my bare feet on our favourite rock and reach into my shoulder bag for the urn. Now that I'm here I don't want to part with him.

I sit for a moment staring out to sea with the urn resting on the yellow and red marbled rock between my feet. Day after day, and then year after year, we made this journey together, to place our footprints on this rock and declare it home. Now mine are the only two damp marks on the dry stone.

I open the urn and stand, reaching my hand out over the water, watching the contents blow away across the undulating surface of the sea.

By releasing him here his ashes can be churned by the waves, to mix with the salt and the sand, as the tide ebbs and flows, brushing our rock, forever home.

Six

Isla - 2017

I unlock the door to my apartment as the taxi drives away. Inexplicably, my longed-for sanctuary feels empty. The beautiful, private place that I've created, which normally gives me such peace after a long day at work, is now an alien space.

Whilst I was in Scotland, I couldn't wait to return and get on with my life. I was frustrated by how much my parents' life had been on a repeating loop. Never stepping towards the new. Now that I've left their world behind, I find that I miss the old worn carpets and the very particular smell of their home. In truth. I miss them.

If I'm honest, all that bluster and exasperation was self-justification. Frustration with them over their lifestyle choices, prevented me from dwelling on my own.

I needn't have been so caught up with work. I could have accepted Mam's anxiety, phobia, pig-headed-stubbornness, whatever it was, instead of trying to change her.

I hang up my coat and put my shoes in the cupboard under the bench seat before carrying my suitcase to the bedroom to unpack.

Most items go automatically into their set positions in the mirrored wardrobe, but I need to find homes for the items that I bought in West Kilbride. These clothes seem so out of step with the person who lives in this apartment, but I want to keep them. I'm changing.

In the past I would have left them in Scotland, for use whilst I was there, and then donated them to charity. But here they are, in Dortmund. These clothes suggest leisure time. My subconscious is finally shifting its priorities.

The quality sleep - that I predicted would arrive with a return to my beautiful *wide* bed - has failed to materialise. Instead, I lie staring up at the ceiling, ruminating on the change that is coming to life here in Dortmund. I'm no longer my only consideration. I have a dependent.

Isla - 2017

I'm not sure what's wrong with me but I'm concerned. The ghost of Mam's dementia is hovering again, unspoken in the dark recesses of my mind. I haven't even made it through my first week back. My secretary set up my habitual five meetings before lunch and I've had to reschedule two of them.

My ability to read and retain information from the documents piling up on my desk is no better. The hyper-focus that I am used to is gone. Other thoughts keep intruding, as I scan the papers. I'm supposed to be hitting the ground running, to catch up with everything that I missed whilst I was away. This is a disaster.

I made it to the end of the week and had a couple of days in bed. But that seems to have made things worse. I feel more lethargic than ever.

I knock on Peter's door, opening it as he calls for me to enter.

'Isla! Please sit down. What can I do for you?'

I very rarely have any problem that I can't sort out for myself, so he's not used to me requesting to see him.

'I'm concerned. I'm not keeping up with my workload. I don't think I will make the deadline at the end of the week unless I can delegate some of my tasks to the rest of the team.'

'I saw from the diary that you've been rescheduling quite a lot of meetings since you returned.'

I'm mortified. He knows. I should have guessed he would find out. He runs a tight ship, and nothing slips past him.

However, I'm stunned by his next words.

'I'm not at all surprised. Grief expresses itself in many ways. It's a complicated set of emotions. So often, they catch up with us once the first emergency has been dealt with.'

'You think this is grief?'

'What are your symptoms?'

'Muscle aches - but no flu symptoms or exercise to explain them, poor concentration, lethargy, break-through thoughts, loss of appetite.'

'Given your recent experiences, I think grief is a likely explanation. My wife described the same, and of course you are experiencing a double loss. It's not just your father, it's your mother too.'

I can feel my core locking up as Peter speaks.

'Although she is physically still with you, the woman who would have comforted you, and shared your pain at this time, is gone.'

Despite the compassion in his voice, I am deeply embarrassed. This is not the relationship we have had historically. I know that he means well.

He is a kind man. But he only learned about Mam's dementia because there were times when Da needed to speak to me during work hours. He then got the full story when Da died, as I needed to take so much time off.

I am utterly averse to being portrayed or perceived as vulnerable. It is not his deliberate intent. However, this is exactly what he succeeds in doing when he continues.

'It is immensely sad that you have lost your mother to this awful condition.' His sympathetic look is almost more than I can bear, as my true vulnerability is undermining me from within.

'I've lost her, haven't I?' I finally acknowledge.

I can feel my jaw start to shake. I pull my shoulders back and take a firm grip on myself. No crying at work! I can't risk the *emotional, flaky female* label.

Taking a deep breath, I say resolutely.

'So, what can I do? It's interfering with my work.'

'Isla you can't *do* anything. You have to allow yourself to *be,* to *feel*. You must let time pass whilst you begin to *accept* what has happened, and gradually *adjust* to your new situation.'

'But what about my responsibilities here?'

'As you suggested, we will need to delegate some of your workload until you feel able to resume your normal duties.'

Peter is being incredibly kind, but I'm deeply ashamed. You can't have one of your top executives running at half measures and expect to succeed in business. That is not the model I have worked to all my life. However right now, I don't seem to have any choice in the matter.

The one thing I still have control over is my ability to improve my communication with Mam. Learning French is a top priority. So, this evening I am at the dining table with my laptop, listening and repeating my sentences about ordering coffee, and simultaneously researching dementia.

Whilst I've known for a few years that Mam has mixed dementia, which in her case is vascular dementia with Alzheimer's, I have never faced up to what this will mean for her long-term.

As I search for symptoms that fit Mam's experience, I come across something called fronto-temporal dementia. I wonder if she might have this too, as it impairs a person's use of language. Perhaps it could be an explanation for Mam speaking French? However, reading on it seems to be more of a difficulty using language to express oneself.

As I continue to scan the pages another type catches my attention. Posterior cortical atrophy, it sounds awful. The cells at the back of the brain, which interpret what the eyes see, are damaged. The eye sees but the brain doesn't understand.

This sounds a bit similar to my experience when Da died. Preparing for that meeting, my brain refused to interpret what I was looking at. But, of course, that was because my full attention was elsewhere.

Evidently, this problem is a symptom of Alzheimer's disease. As well as a condition in its own right. I wonder if this is what was happening to Mam as she looked at the photographs. She had after all been shaking her head and looking confused.

From what I've gleaned here, it's not like being blind - where limited information passes from the eye to the brain. Instead, there is plenty of information arriving but chaos in the interpreting mechanism.

The more I think about it, the more I think this must be what Mam is experiencing. How utterly terrifying.

My muddle-headedness in recent weeks has added to my concern for my own future, however, the science of heritability in dementia seems to be uncertain. There are definitely rare genetic forms that are proven to be heritable, but much to my relief the familial links seem to be more tangled up with environmental factors for the others.

Perhaps it's better not to know what's coming.

Seven

Isla - 2017

I unlock the front door of my parent's house. It smells musty. No one has been inside for a couple of months. I should have thought about asking a neighbour to pop in here too, to open the windows from time to time, but to be fair, I hadn't intended to be away this long when I returned to Germany.

Life in Dortmund has been all consuming, especially since I started feeling more like my normal self at work. I still fear juggling regular visits for Mam, with preparing everything for the new merger, but I am trying.

I have created a new role for a permanent assistant to share my workload. He started last week and it's already making a difference. I am no longer pulling other team members off task. I feel guilty at the extra expense, but Peter has pointed out that anyone else in my role would have taken an assistant a long time ago. If only to work an acceptable number of hours a week and have time off for holidays. How did I not notice what an utter control freak I've been?

Thanks to my new assistant, I am here now, but it really isn't practical for me to be away from the office too often. There I go again. I really do seem to believe that I am the only person capable of making a difficult decision.

I move from room to room throwing open the windows, and as the kettle boils, I sit down to make a list of tasks. I need to organise putting the house on the market.

It will be sad to say goodbye to my parental home, but to be honest, I did my separating decades ago. Beyond my attachment to my parents, my remaining sentiments are for the village and the coastline rather than this house.

The truth is that I feel more German than British these days, although I'm not sure what will happen for people in my position as the UK government goes ahead with Brexit.

If the house here is to be sold, then everything must go. My apartment in Germany is already full, and my parents and I have very different tastes in possessions.

I've brought a spare suitcase for photographs, and maybe there will be the odd souvenir from my childhood, but otherwise Cancer Care on Main Street are going to be huge beneficiaries from the sixty years that my parents lived their settled life in the village.

I might as well start as I mean to go on. I place the empty suitcase on the low coffee table in the front room ready for books. However, as I take the first one off the shelf, I lower myself to the sofa, and begin to turn the pages.

It belonged to Da. A book about sailing that he must have bought in the 1960s. The style of cover and the printing methods don't allow it to be any more recent.

What am I doing? If I stop and read each one before putting it in the case, I'll be here all night. This task is obviously going to be harder than I first thought. Each item stands for so much about my parents. There just isn't time. I need to drop these off in the morning on my way to visit Mam.

I can't wait to share my unexpected new language skills with Elspeth and Adjavella. Despite being frantic with work I have continued to find time for my French course. I've listened and repeated basic phrases and sentences every morning whilst eating my breakfast, and again every evening whilst lying in the bath.

I'm not yet proficient, but as time is of the essence, I've focussed on words that will be useful for chatting with Mam, assuming she's not still speaking that strange dialect.

I arrive at Suncrest wheeling my empty suitcase with a spring in my step.

'Guess what?' I say to Adjavella with a huge grin, even before I've said hello. 'I should be able and give you some proper time off! I've been learning French. I'm doing quite well with general day-to-day things, so I'll be able to have real conversations with Mam.'

For some reason Adjavella's not showing the warmth and relief at this news that I had expected. She glances across at Elspeth before replying.

'Isla, I'm so sorry, Tilly's health has declined considerably in the last few weeks, and she isn't really speaking anymore.'

I feel utterly deflated. I had such high hopes for long conversations with Mam.

Adjavella tries to reassure me.

'Tilly still understands French when I speak to her, so there's a chance that you will be able to reach her. She'll hear what you're saying, and know that you want to communicate with her, even if she doesn't reply.'

Elspeth can see that I'm disappointed.

'It's wonderful that you found the time to learn! I'm afraid I haven't, so all the responsibility is still falling to Adjavella. I'm sure Tilly will be delighted to hear someone else speaking her language. Why don't you go through and surprise her?' she suggests with a gentle ushering movement of encouragement.

Adjavella and I head down the corridor together. As we walk, she tries to add another layer of encouragement and reassurance.

'I think your mother will be very happy that someone besides me is speaking a language that she understands. She's developed the habit of looking past the English-speaking care staff, as if they don't exist. I think she knows that they're not a useful source of information. I'm sure your French will elicit a very different response.'

Mam is lying on her bed when we enter her room. Adjavella pulls an upright chair up close to the pillows, and I swing an armchair around to sit at her feet.

I take a deep breath and tentatively begin.

'Bonjour Tilde.'

She will only become confused if I call her Mam.

'Je m'appelle Isla.'

Mam looks across at me but there's no other response.

Adjavella, with her much better accent, tries to engage Mam in our conversation.

'Tilde, Isla is your daughter, she's come to visit you from Germany.'

The reaction is electric but it's not the type we had hoped for. Mam becomes completely rigid. It's as if she's turned to stone.

Adjavella quickly leans forward to check that she's breathing.

Neither of us have a clue what's going on.

Tilde - 2017

'She's come to visit you from Germany'.
It's happened. I always said it would and no one believed me.
They've come for me now.
Hide.
Maman! Papa!
Hooves, … guns, … hide. … SILENCE!
Go.
Walking, … walking.
Houses, … windows, … people.
Walking, … walking.
Come on quickly.
Engines, … motorbikes,
Hide, … hide!
Walking, … walking, … walking.
Stations, … parklands,
Walking, … walking.
Heavy … bags … sore arms,
Walking, … walking.

Isla - 2017

Eventually Mam's body relaxes, but what follows is worse to see. Mam starts crying and calling out. Increasingly agitated, she thrashes around and becomes entangled in her bedding.

Adjavella tries to reassure her and sometimes it seems to be working, but then her distress returns. I'm just standing at the foot of her bed looking on. I feel utterly powerless to help. When Mam stuffs her hand into her mouth in an attempt to silence herself, it is more than I can bear. I feel as if my own heart will break.

She is obviously having some kind of flashback. It's quite clear that the event she's re-living is more distressing than anything I've ever known.

Eventually Mam is calm and Adjavella indicates that we should leave. We return to reception.

'What just happened?' I ask, taking a seat, as my legs are a little shaky.

'I have no idea.' Adjavella admits perching on the edge of the desk. 'Something I said had a strong impact. Like it was traumatic. Did you catch what she said?'

'I heard something about parks, and gardens, but shouldn't those be happy memories? There was something about horses too, I think.'

'Mm. She also mentioned your grandmother telling her stories so that she wouldn't be scared. And something about walking on a long journey. This is just a thought but … is it possible she could have been a refugee? One of those escaping during the German invasion?'

I feel sick.

'You said that I'd just come from Germany, didn't you? Was that the trigger?' Have I been repeatedly triggering my mother for decades with every mention of the place that I call home?

'Possibly.' Adjavella crosses to sit beside me.

'If … if she experienced life under the Nazis, that could explain why she was so furious when I wanted to go to Germany to study. Why didn't she tell me? I don't understand.'

Confused, I twist around so that I can look at Adjavella.

'There wasn't a trace of a French accent in her English. Why would she go to such lengths to hide her childhood?'

Adjavella rests a comforting hand on my knee.

'I'm afraid that's something Tilly can't explain to you anymore. Do you have other family you can ask?'

'No.' I say slumping back into my chair. 'She and I are the last.'

I need space. To feel close to Da. I can't deal with this crazy rewriting of history on my own. I feel as if I have a large boulder in my abdomen.

I head out along the coast towards Portencross. The old castle is closed but there is still plenty of daylight. This fortified building with the canon at its base is a reminder that people have been at war for thousands of years.

Battles have left marks on the landscape all around me. Here it's possible to study the ruins, and piece together the facts. Unfortunately, a different war has left a deep imprint on my mother's psyche, and I have no way to find out what happened, or to help ease her torment.

Why on Earth didn't she confess that her past was at the route of her resistance to my taking up German? I had thought that it was a resistance to me studying a foreign language in general, on the grounds that it would encourage me to travel and leave home. I never considered any other language, so it never occurred to me that she might have had a different response if I had come home wanting to study Spanish or Danish.

It's unbearable to think of the pain I must have caused her. Although I don't regret the decision for myself. The Germany that I know is very different from the Nazi regime of Mam's past, and the country has given me every opportunity, and a great life.

However, had I known the truth, I could have trodden more gently, instead of criticising Mam for her parochial ways.

Tilly - 1978

Tilly is standing in the kitchen with her back to her daughter, stirring white sauce for the fish pie. Her fingers, where she is gripping the wooden spoon, are as white as the sauce she is making, and she has never used such force to prevent the flour catching on the bottom of the pan.

If she turns now, in response to Isla's sarcastic tone, and accusations of narrow-mindedness, she knows that she will say too much. Better to allow her daughter to think her small-minded and insular, than that Isla has her eyes opened to the pain and devastation that they can bring.

For once James is not helping. He is encouraging Isla in this horrendous plan to immerse herself in their language, to set her sights on a career in the very country that tried to engulf and annihilate her homeland.

It feels like such a betrayal. They speak about progress and expansion. Partnerships and collaborations. International agreements and educational opportunities. But they just don't know what those people are capable of, and how insidious their methods can be.

It seems that the only way to convince her daughter to take another course, would be to admit that she has been lying to Isla about her origins for the last fourteen years.

On this point, Tilly has not changed her mind, nor will she ever. The whole complex story of her past must remain a secret. The Germans tried to take everything, but they will not get her daughter, and they will not get her own peace of mind.

Isla - 2017

I take a seat astride the canon, like I used to as a tiny child. Mam would often sit right behind me, holding me in place, whilst Da stood in front, to take our photo, or simply admire the two people he loved, having fun together. For in the early days, Mam and I had delighted in each other's company.

If only she had been willing to teach me French at home, our bond could have been unbreakable. The surge of regret flowing through me is devastating. Mam is obviously such a skilled linguist. Why couldn't she see that my wish to learn German was that same passion for languages?

As far as I can tell, Mam spoke both English and French without a trace of a foreign accent, which suggests that she learned them both when she was very young. That she can also speak a rare dialect is a further sign of the time she spent in France before she met Da.

Mam has always hated to talk about her past. When I was about eight years old, I wanted to know about my grandparents, and pressed her until she told me that her father died when she was very young, and that her mother had not been around much. She said that this was why she'd been so happy to meet Da. Once the two of them got married he, and later I, became her world.

She had always been adamant. Look forward, never back.

I had respected this at the time, and Mam's stubborn streak meant that I knew better than to bring it up again. However, the more scraps of information I uncover, the more I wish that I had pressed her for further details.

It's hard to imagine what line of work would have taken a young Renfrewshire couple to France at such a troubled time, particularly with a small child in tow.

Of course, the Tilde family origins in Renfrewshire could have all been misdirection on Mam's part. Although without Scottish parents it's hard to explain how she came to speak fluent English with a Scottish accent.

I feel as though, with every passing minute, I know less and less about my background.

I'm still troubled by whether Da knew any of this. It would have been a huge ordeal to bear such trauma alone. However, I've seen enough of Mam's determination to know that she's capable of anything she sets her mind to. In fact, the only reason that I'm learning anything now, is because her mind and her iron will are no longer working together.

This thought fills me with discomfort. It's almost voyeuristic to uncover information that she would never voluntarily share. As was witnessing her experiencing deep pain when she is normally such a private person.

The dementia has robbed her of both her free will, and her dignity.

Eight

Isla - 2017

I head straight to the care home from the airport. This is a flying visit but such a necessary one, as it is almost five weeks since I was last in Scotland. I will see Mam tonight and again first thing in the morning but then I must be on the 10am train back to Glasgow.

Apart from a washbag and a change of clothes, my suitcase is full of papers that I shall review during my layover at Luton on Sunday. I have a meeting with the finance team from the bank on Monday, and I need to be word perfect.

Elspeth is behind the desk in reception when I arrive, I'm almost afraid to enquire about Mam.

'There's been a lot of change since you were last here.'

My heart sinks. Not again.

'She's been trying to leave and growing angry and upset that we're keeping her here against her will.'

This is a horrible thought. Mam has always been so calm and contented here when I've visited, and she and Adjavella have formed such a close relationship.

'She was happy with us when your father was visiting, and she knew who he was. Now, with her mind dwelling on the past, and without any real conversation with us, she is responding less and less to her actual surroundings. Adjavella has been doing her best to stimulate conversation, and Tilly does occasionally initiate contact, but it's always with memories from way back in her own childhood. We took her out for some fresh air in the local area, but she showed no sign of recognising where she was.'

'But she's lived in West Kilbride for sixty years, how can she not recognise it?'

'Isla, I'm sorry, but Tilly's dementia has really progressed in the last month. Very little is making sense to her.'

I'm consumed with despair, and I can't stop my eyes from welling up. I wheel my suitcase across the room to the chairs and sit, head bent, resting my forehead on the handle. I don't want Elspeth to see my tears.

However, Elspeth, aware of my distress, comes over to sit with me.

'Mam must be so frightened,' I blurt.

'It *is* terrifying. I promise you, we're all doing our best for her, and trying to find things she enjoys. Adjavella has found some beautiful coffee-table books written in French. And some others mainly with illustrations. They spend lots of time looking at them.'

As we speak, Adjavella enters via the internal door carrying an illustrated book about gardens.

'Hi Isla, Tilly and I have just come back from a walk around the garden, so I thought this book might be a good one.'

I hesitate, worried after the response that I triggered last time I visited.

'It's ok,' Adjavella spots my reluctance. 'I can come with you if you like. I left Tilly's coat over the back of one of her chairs by mistake. It will give me a chance to hang it up.'

'And don't forget you've got the book to keep her attention away from bad memories.' Elspeth adds.

I truly hope that it works. I'm not sure that I can cope with witnessing that level of distress again.

'Although much of Tilly's past is gone, she usually understands what happens in the room…' Elspeth reassures me, '… as long as she's not too tired. You'll know if she's had enough because she'll become more confused.'

Adjavella gently presses the book into my hand. It's beautiful, and my mind fills immediately with the appropriate French vocabulary.

'Actually, Adjavella,' I square my shoulders to help myself believe what I'm about to say. 'My French is improving and I'm fairly certain I will be ok on my own. I think I need a little mother-daughter time.'

'Of course, I'll be right here if you want me.'

'Wait a minute.' Elspeth says as she rummages in her desk draw. 'Another thing, Tilly likes is having her hair brushed. It calms her down. Maybe you can give that a try too?'

She reaches towards me with a hairbrush, some small hair clips covered in flowers, and a large clip with a huge rose on it. Mam is going to love these.

Unfortunately, when I arrive in Mam's room things are not quite as Adjavella described. Mam is back in her overcoat and currently trying to exit the room via the window.

Tilde - 2017

Tilde spots her coat hanging over the back of her chair. It must be time to go out. It's a bit difficult to find the armholes but she manages to pull it on. She tries the zip, but it's too fiddly. She's warm enough. In fact, she's too hot. She crosses to the window. Perhaps she can get some air.

Tilde stands looking through the glass at the garden. Other people are sitting on benches. If she pulls on the frame it should open. Nothing happens. She pulls harder. It still won't move. It won't move … it won't move! She rattles the glass.

Someone places a hand gently on her shoulder and guides her firmly away towards the table. There's a book in front of her chair, with a picture of a garden on the front. Tilde likes gardens. She opens the book to take a look.

Beautiful flowerbeds. Bright colours.

The woman is touching her hair. She's saying something. What is it? She's going to do her hair. That's nice. The brush feels good. The woman's voice is friendly. Tilde likes it here.

There's a flower on the table. Has it fallen out of the book? She turns the page to see if it's missing. … She reaches out to touch the flower. It feels funny. Not real. There's metal. The woman says it's to go in her hair.

Tilde loses interest. She can feel the woman's hands in her hair, parting the strands. Is she making plaits?

There are twigs on the table too. The woman reaches out and takes one. There's a little jab against her scalp. … Tilde starts. … What's she doing? … The woman apologises.

Tilde returns her attention to the book. The images start to swirl and fragment. It's scary. She can't tell what she's looking at, or how far away the images are. Sometimes the colours rush towards her, and sometimes there is nothing there at all.

Tilde grips the arm of the woman sitting next to her. … Maybe she will keep her safe.

Isla - 2017

I don't know whether it's the result of standing in unaccustomed, prolonged proximity with Mam - so close that I'm bathed in her once familiar scent - or the childhood actions of my hands parting her hair. But suddenly, I'm back in my family home. Sitting on a cushion, on the floor in front of the fire. Mam is sitting on a chair behind me, brushing out my wet hair after my bath.

The memory fades to be replaced by another. Standing in the kitchen before school, waiting for my toast to pop. Asking Mam for the latest must-have hairstyle for the playground.

The atmosphere in the room feels just as it did when I was little. My eyes fill with tears. I associate hairstyling with so many of the close moments with Mam across the decades.

When I was five or six years old, I had a thick rubber swimming-cap with a chinstrap, designed to keep my head warm if it was windy, and to reduce the salt getting into my hair when I played in the sea.

It was always a real fiddle to get on, but Mam developed a speedy ritual. Four long swipes with the brush, before making a quick twist and wrapping motion to create a bun on the top of my head. I would hold this in place whilst she lowered the cap over the top. Instant, loving, and effective teamwork. What went wrong?

I'm glad for this opportunity to try and make her feel special and cared for, in the way that she did for me when I was younger. Although she hasn't said anything, I can feel the contentment in her body as I touch her, and that means a lot.

I'm on my way out when I see Elspeth coming towards me down the corridor. I pause as I open the door to the reception area and hold it open for her to catch up with me.

'How are you Isla?' she asks as she passes me. 'I've not had a chance to check in with you recently?'

'Oh, that's kind of you to ask.' I respond.

This is a golden opportunity. I need to be brave.

As Elspeth approaches her desk, the dam on my anxiety bursts.

'Can I get your professional opinion?' I ask, in a hesitant undertone.

Startled, she pauses and turns to look back at me.

'Of course, what's worrying you?'

'I'm concerned about myself. Do you think I could be following in Mam's footsteps?'

'Oh, I doubt it. Why do you think that? Your mother was well into her seventies before she started having difficulties.'

I let the magnetic door close behind me.

'It's just that I put some documents in the lining of my suitcase for safe keeping and forgot all about them for weeks.'

'That's not unusual.'

'It is for me.'

'Well, at your age it's much more likely to be menopause related.' Elspeth says cheerfully. 'Oestrogen is involved in memory formation. Levels drop significantly in women during menopause, so they often experience short term memory loss.'

'You mean it might not be dementia?'

I'm overcome with emotion. Leaning back against the door, I slide slowly down to the ground. Holding my head in my hands I start to cry. Elspeth squats down beside me and rests her hand on my shoulder.

'Just the menopause.' I'm almost laughing. 'I hadn't even considered that. I'm so relieved. I didn't know how terrified I was, until just now. Thank you so much.'

'Oh, love. How long have you been worrying like this?'

'Three months probably. Since Da died. It's just been niggling away in the back of my mind.'

Elspeth helps me to stand.

'Well, you should definitely have a chat with your doctor, but my gut feeling is menopause.'

Nine

Isla - 2017

In a bid to address the issue of my social isolation, and my complete inability to improve my mid-week work-life balance, I have accepted Peter's invitation to dinner. I am a little unclear as to whether this is with his whole family, or just him and his wife. I know that he has two children, but I can't remember whether they are girls or boys, or even how old they are.

I have no idea why I said yes.

I ring the doorbell and to my horror it's Peter's wife Irena who answers.

'Peter is putting the boys to bed. It's the only time that he sees them during the week, so he may be a little while. Come in. We can have a drink and get to know each other.'

Although Peter and I have worked closely together for years, Irena and I have only met on a handful of occasions at work functions, and to be brutally honest I could never be bothered to invest the time in someone I was unlikely to see for a further year.

I am therefore blindsided when she hands me a glass of wine and says,

'I imagine your father's death must have been devastating for your mother. Did it accelerate her dementia? We were totally unprepared for the effect of my uncle's death on his wife.'

I'm flabbergasted. How can she go straight to such personal questions and deep revelations about her own life with a total stranger? I've only just walked through the door. I glance hopefully towards the staircase but the sounds of squealing and splashing coming from upstairs suggest that Peter will be sometime.

Then the penny drops. I've been set up. Peter has deliberately invited me early so that his wife can talk to me alone.

I wait for the outrage to fire through my system, but to my surprise it never comes. It turns out, that the idea of talking to this warm and solicitous young woman is actually very appealing. She genuinely wants to help, and on top of that, she's had experience of some rather similar situations with relatives.

'Did your aunt have dementia?' I ask experimenting with what it feels like to reach across the barrier of unfamiliarity.

'Mm, Alzheimer's, but only very mildly when my uncle was diagnosed with cancer. She had managed his personal care right to the end with a little help from a community nurse who supervised his medications, but within four months of his death she was in residential care.'

'I don't know if it's the separation from my father, but the speed of Mam's decline over the last three months has really surprised me. Even during the course of those first few weeks, whilst I was organising the funeral, she lost her ability to dress herself. Buttons and zips became a real challenge, and there's now no chance that she can select her own outfits. She doesn't really understand what items are necessary, let alone what might look nice together. It's heart-breaking, as Mam always took such great care over her appearance.'

'That breakneck speed is the shock, isn't it? It feels like, in an instant, the person you know vanishes. My aunt was only sixty when she was diagnosed. She'd been running the office for a major haulage company. I had spoken to her at a Christmas party about retirement plans, and when I visited her the following Easter, not only had she taken early retirement on medical grounds, but she had become completely incapable of managing her own life.'

I think back to the year, or more, during which Da coped alone at home, before Mam needed that level of care.

'Wow, that's fast.'

'I agree,' Irena nods. 'Her situation was unusual. Every person, and every brain is different. That's why we all feel so alone. No one has walked in our shoes before, no one can tell us what to expect.'

There's such lonely truth in her words.

'For me, the worst aspect is Mam's inability to recognise me. She hasn't done so since Da died. In the beginning she did at least know that she had a daughter, and that I was called Isla. She just expected me to be a small child.'

'Oh, that's hard. You're there in the room, but you won't do.'

'That's it exactly. Back then there was still quite a lot of the old Mam present. So, I kept thinking that I would be able to reason with her, explain who I was, and that she would remember.'

'Did it ever work?'

'No. Not really. My only consolation is that her carer says Mam is calmer with me than she is with unfamiliar people. So perhaps I smell right or something. Maybe her subconscious has a sense of family, even if the rest of her mind is none the wiser.'

'Well as a parent, I think it is entirely possible that you would recognise your own child on an animalistic level, even if your conscious mind was struggling. I definitely know the smell of my boys. It makes my stomach flip every time I think about it.'

A look of incredible tenderness and love passes across Irena's face, and just for a moment I have faith that Mam too will know who I am from my smell.

'How mobile is she?' Irena asks. 'You mentioned that your mother can't dress herself anymore.'

'Oh, she moves around her room quite freely, although her walking has become more like a shuffle. She doesn't venture alone into the rest of the care home anymore.'

'Do you think she's frightened of not being able to find her way back?'

'I hadn't really thought about that. She certainly has trouble recognising things at a distance.'

I hear a noise behind me.

'Well look at you two chatting away as if you've been friends forever.'

I smile, as I give Peter a look that will leave him in no doubt, that he has been caught in the act. But caught in the act of what? Being kind?

I'm so glad that he invited me tonight. Irena is lovely, and I have high hopes that she might turn out to be the first person here in Dortmund that I can call a friend.

It's the middle of the night and once again I am staring at my ceiling, desperate for sleep. Insomnia has never been a problem before, despite the pressures of work. I suspect that I'm just struggling to adjust to my new circumstances.

The changes in my life are coming thick and fast. Both within me, and within my schedule. It feels good to be spending regular time with Mam.

My whole perspective on our past together has shifted, now that I know her problem was with Germany, and not with me. If only I had known. Everything could have been different.

I could have looked for a job somewhere that didn't upset her so much, and I wouldn't have stayed away during my early twenties when her refusal to visit had felt so personal to me. We could have had three decades of a proper mother-daughter relationship, which have now been lost forever.

I'm desperate for a way to process these huge emotions, but there is no solution. I can't apologise, because Mam doesn't know who I am, or understand the events of our shared past. I can't start from now and build a good relationship going forward, because she can no longer connect with anyone.

I can't understand her through the eyes of someone else and with the benefit of hindsight, because Da is dead and I doubt anyone else would have known her well enough to know her secrets.

I'm a mess of unresolved feelings.

Ten

Isla - 2017

It's seven in the morning. Da was the only person to call me at this time. I hold my breath as I press the button to answer. Given the time difference to the UK I fear the worst.

'Isla, I've got some bad news,'

My heart has surely skipped a beat.

'Tilly has picked up an infection.'

I exhale. Thank God, she's not dead.

'Late November always seems to bring bugs, doesn't it?' I commiserate as the feeling of relief floods through me.

'I agree it's very hard to avoid infections at this time of year. Unfortunately, it's not just a cold. Tilly's developed pneumonia, and so far, she's not responding to the antibiotics. I know you aren't due for another week, but I think you need to come now.'

'How did she contract the pneumonia? She barely sees anyone?'

'It's not an infection brought on by contact with others.' Elspeth explains, kindly. 'People with dementia often have problems swallowing, and accidentally inhale food or drink. That then causes a problem in their lungs.'

I've definitely seen Mam do that. Lots of scary coughing and gasping for breath.

'Unfortunately, the dementia itself can mean that the body fails to recognise the need to activate the immune system to fight the infection.'

Wow, this is serious. I want Da. How ridiculous.

I can't lose them both in under six months! How can this be happening? She was fine when I last saw her. Confused but physically in good health. Our family are tough. We get up and get on with it. We've all been lucky. It's never been just about mental attitude. We've all been blessed with incredibly resilient constitutions. Come on Mam. Fight.

I can't believe it. Whichever route I try to plan, one leg is fully booked. Perhaps if I take a train to Dusseldorf and fly from there instead. That works. OK, there's a flight into Gatwick and a connection up to Glasgow. Damn!

I hit the table beside my computer with such force, that I have to tuck my palm under my armpit, to gain relief from the pain.

It's happened again. The Glasgow flight from Gatwick is fully booked. I'm running out of time. I need to leave in twenty minutes if I'm to catch the train to Dusseldorf.

There is a flight to Edinburgh that has a seat. Done. I will just have to take a taxi for the final bit. That will be one happy driver.

Isla - 2017

I'm on one of the last flights to land, and Edinburgh airport is almost empty. I just hope there are still taxis at the rank because I ran out of time to book one. I power walk along beside the shuttered shops, the wheels of my suitcase thundering along behind me. The sound ricochets around the empty terminal making me feel very conspicuous.

Three taxis, two people, I'm going to be ok.

'West Kilbride please.'

'You know you're in Edinburgh? That's a heck of a way from here.'

'My only choice,' I say ruefully. 'Mam's dying. As we speak.'

'Oh, lassie, I'm sorry. Jump in. Don't tell anyone. I've got a monitoring system for the speed cameras and police vehicles. We should make good time.'

Those devices may be illegal, but today I don't care. In Germany we're allowed to go as fast as we like on the autobahns, and that's what I need right now.

At Suncrest I ring the bell and a member of the night staff lets me in. I explain who I am, and he ushers me towards Mam's room. I am relieved, and not at all surprised, to see Adjavella sitting on a chair at the head of Mam's bed. She's holding her hand and watching her shallow, laboured breathing by the light of a small lamp on the table behind her.

'It won't be long now,' Adjavella whispers.

I feel a lump forming in my throat.

'I'm so pleased you got here in time.'

She stands.

'Take my chair, I'll give you this time alone together.'

As she steps towards me, I surprise myself by putting out my arms and she steps into them and gives me a brief hug as if it is the most natural thing in the world, before carrying on towards the door.

'Actually, Adjavella …'

I hesitate.

'I'd like a few minutes alone. But, after that, could you come back? I'd really like you to be with us at the end. You've done so much for her, and if she has any awareness left it will give her confidence if you're here as well. To be honest it would be nice for me too.'

I look down at my hands reluctant to confess.

'I've not seen anyone die before.'

Adjavella gives me a sympathetic look.

'Of course, I'll be back in a few minutes.'

I cross to the chair and resume vigil at Mam's side. How am I going to express my deepest feelings, via a language that I still don't really speak?

I agonise for several minutes before realising that it's not about the perfect sentence. What is the important information?

'Tilde, I love you' I say, as I place a gentle kiss on her forehead. There's no point in calling her Mam. She doesn't know who I am.

As I lean over her, I'm delighted to see that the locket I gave her is under her nightgown. Adjavella must have done that today. I doubt Mam sleeps with it on every night. I must thank her. It's obvious that she truly understands what it's like to be far from family and loved ones, especially when they're ill.

I'm holding Mam's frail little bird-like hand as it rests on the covers, when Adjavella slips back into the room. She pulls a second chair up beside me. Then, taking my free hand in hers, she reaches out her other hand and gives Mam's knee a gentle squeeze, creating a circle of support. It's reassuring through the rattling sound of mucus collecting in Mam's throat.

I'm so grateful. We stay in this position until Mam's chest no longer makes its tiny motion towards the ceiling, and I know for certain that it's over.

No more suffering, no more confusion, no more tantalising hope of connection. It has happened. She is gone. I am alone.

Isla - 2017

Mam died at three this morning. I've been in bed for over an hour, with no sign of sleep. All our significant interactions, be they joyful or challenging, are cascading through my mind. Ambushing each other as they rush to the fore.

As memory after memory crowd in, I climb into the attic, seeking evidence of love and connection.

In an ancient suitcase of Mam's clothes, below a thick tweed jacket and long dark overcoat, I find the flimsy diaphanous brown dress, covered in yellow and white circles, that Mam wore to every social event in the seventies. I remember as a small child getting tangled in its sleeves.

Peeking through the sheer material, I spot the bright orange wool of her sixty's jumper dress. Our early photos show me clinging to the hem, but I have no memories of my own.

I pull them both out and hold them to my nose, breathing in deeply, in the vain hope that they smell like Mam. Sadly, the only smell is of mothballs, and I start to cough.

I hold them in my lap as I rummage further.

Towards the bottom of the trunk is a knitted swimsuit. A truly historic garment. The only thing going for it is its colour, which has not faded a bit, across the decades. It is bright red. I can't imagine having to wear such a thing, and I've no idea why Mam has kept it all these years. Now, of course, I can't ask her.

My tears run steadily and smoothly down my cheeks, over my lips, into the corners of my mouth, and on down my chin. I don't try to stop them. I lower my head and let them fall onto the dresses and the memories.

Elspeth and Adjavella look up with a start as I crash through the front door at Suncrest. Speaking at a mile a minute, waving my precious piece of paper.

'It was in a tin box.'

They both look puzzled.

'At the bottom of an old suitcase full of clothes.'

I gasp for breath having run all the way here.

'This was on top of a stack of papers.' I rush on.

I pause for effect.

'Mam may have died Tilly MacLeod of West Kilbride, Scotland, but she was born Clothilde Marec in Paris on the 26th of May 1936!'

They both gasp.

'So, she *was* French!' Elspeth seems a little slow on the uptake this morning. 'It's incredible, her English was so good. I mean her accent wasn't exactly local, but it was most definitely Scottish. I would never have guessed English was her second language.'

'Clothilde, what a beautiful name' Adjavella sighs with delight. 'I wish I could have called her by it. Clothilde Marec, I'm so pleased to have known you.'

Having shared the final piece in the puzzle, the adrenaline, that's been coursing through my body for the last thirty-six hours, suddenly leaves me. I feel nothing but exhaustion.

I cross to the chairs and examine the document more closely.

'This piece of paper …' I turn it over in my hand. 'It's the explanation we've been after. And yet, all I have are questions. And a desperate – sadness.' I swallow hard. 'Sadness that I never really knew my own mother.'

Isla - 2017

I climb the ladder into the attic and look despairingly at the vast array of belongings. I wonder if Elspeth needs anything for the care home.

One corner is piled high with Da's outdoor sports equipment. Perhaps Andrew would like some. Although he seems the kind of man to have his own top-quality gear. I guess this will all go to charity.

What I find most heart-breaking is the enormous quantity of toys and child-sized pieces of furniture awaiting the time when I would give my parents a grandchild.

My childhood cot and highchair, a wooden tricycle, the frame for a three-quarter sized bed, all kept without my knowledge in the hope that they could pass them on.

A whole other life that would have needed a whole other me. I was always destined to grab the wider world with both hands. I think the fact that they never told me this stuff was here shows that deep down my parents knew this too.

Isla - 2017

The house clearance people came with their van this morning and stripped the place, all except for my parents' writing desk which Andrew asked for, and a small dressing table from my parent's room.

It's a sweet little item, and although it doesn't really fit with the scheme in my German apartment, I don't want to part with it. Andrew has agreed to look after it for me until I can organise shipping.

The doorbell rings and he's outside with the boot of his estate car already open.

'I'm fairly certain they're both going to fit.' he says, measuring the spaces against his own arm span.

'Hi Andrew, how are you?'

'Oh, sorry! Fine thank you, fine. Apologies for being in such a rush. We've got a dinner at the golf club later, so I must press on. Come and see me before you go!'

'Will do.' I reply, double checking the size of the available space through the hatchback.

I reach to remove the long slim drawer of the dressing table so that it doesn't fall out as we move it, but it's not empty. Two neatly wrapped packages are staring accusingly at me.

Thank goodness I decided to keep this table myself. These packets could have been lost to a house clearance sale. I take a closer look. One is soft and carefully wrapped in tissue paper. Now is not the time to open it.

The other bundle feels firm, like a stack of letters. They are wrapped in a handkerchief and held together with a piece of string, into which one final letter has been tucked. My father's handwriting is on the envelope.

If these are love letters to my mother, they could have information about her past and give me some idea of how much Da knew. However, no child wants to read the deeply personal elements of their parents' relationship.

'What've you got?' Andrew asks.

'Sadly, no diamonds,' I joke, 'but there are some letters from Da. I'm not sure I'm ready for those.'

'Leave them where they are.' he says cheerfully.

It seems cowardly, but it might be a good solution.

He puts out his hand and squeezes me on the shoulder.

'I won't touch them. You can come back and collect them any time. It will give me a chance to see you.'

I'm so pleased to hear him say this. Despite the slightly blustering persona he is a lovely man and I have a wealth of memories of him and Da together over the years. I like the idea of staying in touch.

Eleven

Isla - 2017

I must admit that when Mam died, I fled. I closed the door on my parents' house, jumped on a plane, and buried myself in work.

My new reality was too awful to face, and self-deception allowed a retreat into my old workaholic pattern.

Luckily, with the focus on the merger, signs of Christmas have been rather absent around the office. I've been frightened of all the Scottish memories they might trigger. Thankfully, I've made it through to lunchtime today, 23rd December, without a public meltdown.

The change in the office to stollen and Christmas biscuits as the accompaniments to coffee over the last month, were the only exceptions in this Christmas-free zone.

Now, with all my colleagues heading off to celebrate with family, this building will be closed until the morning of the 27th, and for the first time I am face-to-face with my orphan status.

Although I have never been one for taking my full annual-leave allowance, I have always been in the habit of spending the time between the 23rd of December and the 2nd of January in Scotland.

Even in the difficult years with Mam I only ever missed one Christmas. The three of us would decorate the house when I arrived on Christmas Eve, and the next day, after a bowl of porridge for breakfast, we would head out for the traditional Christmas Day walk, whatever the weather, whilst the roast cooked slowly in the oven, ready for our return.

Tilly - 1990

Tilly closes the oven door and looks at her watch. 8.30am. All the preparations are done. Christmas dinner is on track and will look after itself whilst they head to Loch Thom for their walk.

She can hear Isla moving around upstairs and is feeling a little apprehensive. The sequence of last night's events has been playing on her mind. If only she had had the power of foresight.

The flight was due to arrive at 10.30pm and James had gone alone to pick Isla up from the airport whilst she stayed behind to finish baking and set up the decorations ready for hanging as soon as they got back.

She had hoped that hanging the decorations together would start the process of mending their relationship, as it's been two years since Isla's last visit home.

Unfortunately, Isla's flight was delayed. There had seemed no harm in climbing into bed to read until they arrived. However, she'd been tired after a busy day and had promptly fallen asleep. She'd been dead to the world until her alarm went off at six this morning.

Why on Earth didn't James wake her when they got back? Now Isla will think that she doesn't care.

Tilly braces herself to meet her daughter at the sound of Isla's footsteps on the stairs.

'Hi Mam. How're you?' Isla's words are friendly enough, but she doesn't cross the room to embrace her mother and instead walks across to the cupboard containing the mugs asking, 'Do you want something?'

Tilly is unsure how to respond. Isla's actions are very cold and disconnected but her words are simultaneously solicitous. Is she cross? Is this just her new way now that she's a business executive? Is she trying to avoid an argument? Would saying something about last night make things better, or worse?

Tilly wants to give her daughter a hug, but she looks so brittle and stand-offish, perhaps now is not the time.

Isla - 2017

There will be no roast for me this year. It's not worth it for one. Instead, I stopped by the delicatessen on the way home last night, and I have a choice of things to nibble on whilst I wait for life to resume.

I know what's coming - as free time gives my darker thoughts free reign - and I accept that it's time to stop running. But I'm not sure that I'm ready to face the onslaught of emotion.

Over the last few weeks, I've had the occasional glimpse, of a totally unexpected rage boiling beneath the surface, only kept in check by my workaholic drive.

I'm so furious with Mam for keeping such a huge secret about her past that I haven't wanted to delve any further. It wasn't just her past that she was denying. It was my ancestry too! I'm half French!

All I know from the birth certificate is that my mother was born in Paris in the tenth arrondissement, and I had two French grandparents. Henri Marec and his wife Camille - who's family name was Guery.

If she had only told me who she was from the beginning, I could have asked her all about them. I could have known what they looked like. Whether like me they enjoyed mathematics and logic problems, or whether they were more like Mam, with her interest in making and creating things and her passion for gardening.

How could she have denied me all this!

With nothing else to do, it is time to explore the suitcase of documents and other objects that I brought back from Scotland last month. The first item that I remove is the biscuit tin, where I found the birth certificate.

As I lift the lid and remove its contents, I'm surprised to find my own ten-yard swimming certificate from my primary school, and a badge to say that I had passed elementary level in gymnastics. I seem to remember that this involved doing a headstand, a handstand, a cartwheel and a bridge, nothing to threaten the Olympic team.

Mam had been deeply immersed in my life in the early years, really supportive and interested. Then suddenly it all changed when I hit puberty at fourteen. I thought perhaps she couldn't handle me growing up, but now I'm sure it had more to do with me choosing to study German for O-grade.

If only she'd told me the truth. I saw deep terror in the room that day at Suncrest. Terror and unimaginable grief. And yet I have no accompanying words of explanation. No clues as to what happened.

Did she experience something directly? Did she see some horrific event? Or was it prolonged anxiety - the background fear of what might happen - that penetrated deep into the psyche of my infant mother?

It is so insignificant in comparison, but this not knowing has been enough to mess with my peace of mind.

The next item I find is my mother's personal address book. It has very few addresses and even fewer phone numbers. There are a couple of names that I recognise, women from the village, long-term friends of my mother, whom I spoke to briefly at her funeral.

Much to my delight, many of the staff from the care home had wanted to attend Mam's funeral, and as some of her friends had also had mobility issues, I chose to have Mam's service in a local church for easy access. However, when it came time to go with her coffin to the crematorium, I went alone, leaving Elspeth and Adjavella to host the wake.

I'd returned for the last half hour, but by that time many people had gone, so my contact with Mam's friends that day had been very limited.

Christmas Day is not the day for phone calls, but I add the phone numbers for these women to my to-do list. Mam must have discussed her concerns with them.

All parents express opinions about their children's life choices. If Mam and Da for once disagreed - it was his backing that won-the-day for me - then she must surely have looked outside the family for support. Perhaps these women will be able to fill in just a little of the background.

At the very bottom of the tin are two aged and very delicate looking pieces of paper. I remove them and unfold them carefully onto my lap.

The first is the death certificate of Chloe Guery, who died on the 17th of March 1951, aged 55, in a place called Barantan in the Auvergne region of France.

I wonder if the Camille Guery, from Mam's birth certificate, and this Chloe Guery are the same person. Could one be a diminutive like Tilde, and Tilly for Clothilde? Chloe would have been in her early forties as a mother, but the dates are not impossible.

If this woman is her mother it could explain, perhaps in part, why Mam left France. She would have been almost fifteen when Chloe died. That's young to lose a parent. As a teenager you are still growing and forming your outlook on life. I can attest to the fact that losing your mother shakes you up at any age.

The next document is for a Joseph Guery, also of Barantan. He died a short while earlier in 1948 at the age of 58. I'm a bit confused about who he is. Mam's father was called Henri Marec so this can't be her father.

I scan the rest of the faded document. The death was registered by Chloe Guery, wife of the deceased. OK, so these two are spouses, so perhaps relatives of Mam. I was obviously wrong about Chloe being the same person as her mother Camille. So, if Camille didn't die in 1951, what happened to her?

I return to the documents. Chloe's death was registered by someone named Rory Stewart. That's a surprise. He has to be a Scot, surely, with a name like that. It says that his relationship to the deceased is neighbour.

As far as my limited French can tell, the other column requesting information is for recording each person's occupation, and what I think is the word for farmer, is written on Joseph's.

So, my mother may have a connection with the farming community of the Auvergne. This is taking my explorations in a whole new direction. Adjavellá only heard Mam talk about family in Brittany.

I'm regretting that I left the bundles of letters where they were in that drawer. If only I had brought them to Germany. I've finally developed a passion for the investigation, and now have nowhere else to go.

I look up at the urn that is sitting on my bookshelf. ... Mam. ... As much of a puzzle in death as in life. Without knowing more about her past, I haven't felt able to decide about the placement of her ashes. So, for now, she is here with me. The locket I had made for her is also here, around my neck, and in it a picture of Mam instead of the photograph of me.

The office is still closed, and as I can't bear another day at home, I decide to go for a walk along the Emscher. The river is no longer the open sewer that it once was, and the regeneration works have produced some lovely recreational spaces.

As I walk, my whole life turns over in my mind. If Mam is not Scottish - and I am now fairly certain that the Tildes of Renfrewshire were a crafty piece of misdirection on her part - then fifty percent of me is a complete mystery. I hate the way that this is dismantling me from the inside.

With every cherished memory that I replay in my mind, a part has to be discarded, as no longer true, rather like a tree shedding dead leaves. Previously I felt like a flourishing evergreen. Now, with every thought, I am becoming a skeleton of bare branches about to face a harsh winter.

In desperation I try to focus on the elements within me that haven't changed. Da's family on the MacLeod side. I'm certain that they've been fishermen in Scotland for generations, except of course for his uncle, who joined the navy. Granda met his future wife at a naval dance when he was visiting his brother. Without that meeting, Da wouldn't have existed.

She was a West Country girl visiting her brother, who was also in the navy. Despite all of her own family being in the Southwest, she fell in love and agreed to move to Scotland. Perhaps I got my wish to travel and explore the world from her.

This knowledge of Da's family history - regularly passed on by him, as we walked beside the sea that his family had all loved so much - gives me a feeling of standing on solid ground.

Although our branch of the family has dwindled almost to nothing, I am sure that I have third cousins somewhere in the West Country that I could trace.

However, I'm not sure that you can still call people family if the connections are that remote. Especially if there is no one alive who would remember the ancestors who form the bridge.

Although revisiting my MacLeod history this morning has helped a little, I don't think the feelings of uncertainty will go until I can find more answers about Mam's side of the family. I check the time. It will be half past four in Scotland. Hopefully this is a suitable time to catch Mam's friends.

Four phone calls later and I have no extra information. Not a single bit. Two of the women had not even heard on the village grapevine that Mam was born in France and were totally shocked.

All had said the same thing - that Mam had never spoken to them about her life before I was born - and all knew her to be a home bird. They described her as friendly but preferring the company of her immediate family.

Once again, I am at a dead end. Without any answers, how am I supposed to put this behind me, and move on?

Tilly - 1969

Tilly is at the school gate. She can feel Isla's tiny hand wriggling nervously in her own. Today is a big moment in her daughter's life. Her first day at the main school. Despite it only being a local primary, there are many more children all in one place than Isla has ever seen before, and Tilly is hoping that she won't have any trouble getting her to stay by herself.

There are lots of other women here too, all looking rather similarly anxious. Tilly gets a wave, and a beckoning motion, from the mother of a friend of Isla's. But as she is standing in a group of parents with older children, none of whom Tilly knows, Tilly merely nods and smiles shyly in response.

The thought of going over and joining them is too daunting. They have obviously been friends for years. Although Kirsty is someone that she likes to chat to on the beach whilst their children play, Tilly knows that there is never any room in an established group like that, for someone new.

The bell rings and the children start to file towards the open door. To Tilly's surprise, Isla drops her hand, and without looking back, runs headlong across the playground to begin her day of learning.

Tears well in Tilly's eyes. The contrast between her daughter, and herself, couldn't be starker. The trembling movement she had felt in Isla's hand, had been excitement, not anxiety. Her daughter is a bright, confident, inquisitive child, and she can't wait to get into the classroom.

Isla might not know many of the other children, but she isn't fazed by this, she has no need for social acceptance, so long as she has access to something that stretches her mind.

Unfortunately, she herself, completely lacks this focused shield. Tilly is only too aware of the painful cuts inflicted by social rejection, and is more convinced than ever, that she needs to stick to the plan that she formed when she moved to West Kilbride. She must save her energy and hopes for her family. Locals can be passing acquaintances without creating any negative impact, but she will not allow them to undermine her.

James' parents are people that she can rely on, and although neither of them is in the best of health right now, their little unit of five is perfectly fine for taking on the world.

On the rare occasions that Tilly can't look after Isla when James is at work, his parents will sit with her, and the five of them get together for birthdays, holidays, and boat trips in the summer.

Sadly, there's a question mark over how much longer Douglas will have the boat, as his lungs are really not up to the physical work it requires. His cough started about a year ago. Initially it was a tiny, but regular, puff of escaping air, almost like a cat's sneeze, which accompanied him as he went about his work.

Now, he has to pause every minute or two, and the deep, hacking, phlegmy cough that wracks his body each time, is a certain indication that he is deeply unwell. However, he will not go to the doctor.

Eileen is desperately worried about him and has lost a huge amount of weight herself with all the stress. At least, Tilly hopes that is the cause. Her mother-in-law is disappearing before her eyes. The thought that both of James' parents could be terminally ill at the same time is utterly unbearable.

Surely, she and James couldn't lose all four of their parents before they were forty. It would be so unfair. Alone in the world, just the two of them - and Isla of course. Other people have loved ones around for years. Sitting by the fireside, year on year, sharing memories. Memories. Perhaps they are best forgotten anyway.

Twelve

Isla - 2018

It's March, and I'm very grateful that my parents' house has sold after only four months on the market. I could have dealt with everything remotely, but this is going to be the last time that I can ever enter my childhood home. I needed to come back. To be in West Kilbride to say goodbye.

I am clinging to the smallest elements of my heritage. To anything of which I can be certain. Not just my familial Scottish links through Da, but also the geographical locations that root me to this, the first area that I called home. The importance of landscape has greatly increased now that my human tethers are gone.

It's become clear to me that our belief in our own story can be a key component of how we navigate life. It provides a confident base from which we can step into the unknown. I certainly had no idea at the time that this was a gift I had been given as a child. Nor had I been aware of how I'd used it to become a success in my chosen career.

Now that my story has been torn apart, and called out for the lie that it is, I am questioning my interpretation of every event in my life, and of all that I have built based on these lies.

As there is no furniture at the house. I'm staying in an Airbnb up near the station. I take a slow walk down Main Street, scanning the shops and the side roads as I go. It's quite possible that I will never come back. I hope that's not the case. As just the thought makes the tears flow. But I know myself. I wasn't the best at returning when my parents were alive. How likely am I to make the journey just to reminisce?

I let myself into the house and climb the stairs to my old room. If you stand at the window, with your shoulder pressed hard into the corner on the right, and your head turned so that your ear is totally flat against the glass, you can see the sea. I wonder if there will be another child sleeping in this room, who will discover this very important piece of information.

I hope that the new owners are as happy here as my parents were. The building itself is in bad need of updating. Many of the basic features haven't been altered since the early sixties when they moved in. But the atmosphere is full of love. At least that's how it feels today.

I take a last look in all the other rooms, before locking up and dropping my keys with the agent.

So that's that. No parents. No heritage. No home. It's been an astonishing year.

My next stop is Andrew's house. I am going to collect the letters. A removal firm are coming next week to pack and send the dressing table in a shared shipping container, but I don't trust them with the letters. Those are going to travel safely back to Germany in my hand luggage.

He's just finishing dinner when I arrive and tries to persuade me to stay and have a brandy with him, but I'm too restless. So, with the letters zipped firmly into my handbag, I continue down to the beach.

I can see that once again, I have avoided the opportunity to spend time with someone who might become a friend, but I am desperate for one last walk on the sand, and right now, I am certain that this beautiful landscape will provide me with far more solace than any human can.

I stop on our rock and say hello to Da, and then walk on across the golf course. This time I'm able to take the diversion to where Da died. At this time of night, I have the course to myself.

Andrew gave me an account of Da's last moments a few months ago. His ball had landed in this bunker, which meant that for a moment he was out of sight of the others. The best guess is that his heart stopped when he bent down to get the ball, because they found him collapsed in the sand.

One member of their group knew CPR and started at once when they reached him, whilst Andrew phoned the ambulance. But I know from his GP that it was all too late, even with their prompt action.

Da may have died here, but he's not here anymore. In my mind he's down at the shore. I guess that's because he and I never spent time here together. He took up golf long after I left home.

Perhaps Andrew feels his presence in this place that they shared. In a way, I hope that he does, but for me, our rock with its view of the sea will be where I come to find Da if I'm in Scotland again.

Isla - 2018

Today I have an appointment with Peter for a Professional Development Meeting. Usually, I find these meetings exciting opportunities to hear what Peter has in mind for me, and a chance to pitch my own visions of what I can offer the company.

But this time I'm worried. My heart has not truly been in my work since we completed the company restructuring. I have no new ideas to offer, and I'm not even that curious about Peter's vision.

Peter is peering at me over the top of his glasses as I complete my confession.

'Isla, it's likely that you're just burnt out and need a break. In the two years that you've worked in my team, prior to the death of your parents, I have never known you to take more than the compulsory days holiday.'

I bob my head slightly to acknowledge the truth of this statement, as he carries on.

'More significantly I have just discovered from HR that, had it been possible to carry over the leave allowance from one year to the next, by now, with weekends, you would have been owed over a year of vacation time, from the date ten years ago, when you first joined the company!'

'But I know that I've taken some short breaks now and then.'

I definitely remember a few long weekends.

'Those mini breaks only counted against the time-off-in-lieu you accumulated whilst attending conferences and travelling at weekends for meetings. I should never have allowed this to happen. I'm sorry. You were always so adamant that you didn't need, or want, time off, and there was always something urgent to be completed that would benefit from your presence.'

I'm quite shocked to hear how much leave I gave up, and I instantly convert it into time that I could have spent with Mam and Da. If only I could have properly healed the rift with Mam. We could have just hung out together as we did when I was a child. I could have asked her to remind me how to knit.

When I was ten, she had taken such care teaching me to make a woollen hat for a school project. I'd loved doing it, but I've completely forgotten how to create the stitches.

My regrets with Da are totally different. He and I had always talked of hiring a boat and sailing around the Scottish coast, visiting all the islands, and appreciating our ancestry. I'd always assumed that it would be just the two of us, as Mam always wanted to stay close to home, but now that I know her main reason for avoiding Germany, I think perhaps we might have persuaded her to join us. Especially if it meant that she could stay with Da and remain in Scotland.

Hindsight is a painful thing.

I force my attention back into the room and realise that Peter is still speaking.

'Even without the need for a break, and the devastation of losing both your parents, I've been concerned about how you would feel on completion of this merger.'

I look up surprised.

'Really why?'

Up to this point I have deliberately not shared any of my own concerns with him.

'Isla, not only was this merger everything you've worked for since you joined my team, but it has been evident from the way that you spoke at interview, and your input at all your previous development meetings, that you have always had your sights on an opportunity like this. A chance to prove your capabilities to the world.

Now that your talents have been recognised, your vision for the company has been accepted, and your plan is being put into place. What more is there for you to do?'

I'm stunned. He got there before I'd even opened my mouth. He is completely right. *Job done* is exactly how I feel, but I've been struggling to name it. What does this mean? I love my team and working for Peter. I don't want to lose those relationships and be forced to start again in another company.

After an initial sadness acknowledging the truth of our situation, Peter and I went around the workable solutions three or four times, and eventually came up with a plan.

I will take a break for a month, to refresh my tired body and brain, and allow my subconscious time to consider my long-term future. Peter and I will then have another Professional Development Meeting on my return to see where I stand.

I'm very grateful to Peter and my other senior colleagues for taking on extra supervisory roles. I'm delegating many things to my new assistant, and I've accepted that I have to postpone the start of a couple of projects.

I know how lucky I am. The thought of so many unstructured days scares me, but I only have one way that I want to spend this time.

My flight is booked. Next Thursday I will be in Paris! I've no idea where Barantan is, but I'm sure I can solve that with a hire car and a satnav.

Before I leave, I need to face Da's letters. The outer wrapping isn't the mass-produced handkerchief I'd expected. Instead, it's a square of white linen with beautifully embroidered edges. Inside are several pieces of fine airmail paper, of a kind that I haven't seen for decades.

They are covered in my father's tight, neat, handwriting. Interspersed with these are postcard-sized pieces of much thicker paper, each one with the same message in the centre *From James, with all my love!* Followed by the date of one wedding anniversary after another.

However, it's the reverse sides that hold my interest. Each one is a hand painted watercolour scene. The locations are extremely familiar from my childhood, and it is wonderful to see the detail that Da has managed to include. There is no doubt at all that he is the artist, as I recognise his style.

He didn't paint often, as there was not much light after work, but whenever we took family holidays, he would bring his pocket watercolour set and sketch pad. What I remember most though, is his special drawing pencil. I got into so much trouble when I borrowed it for other purposes and destroyed the tip.

There are a few places that I don't recognise, and all look as though they've been painted at around the same time on pages torn from a book.

Tilly - 1958

Tilly and James are at West Kilbride station. He has his arms around her as she stands in front of him, looking up into his face.

'Where are we going? Come on you have to tell me.' She says, tugging at the bottom of his jacket, as she nudges his shoulder encouragingly.

'No, it's a surprise,' he says, chuckling as he shakes his head. 'All I can tell you is that it is one of my favourite places, and if you're to become Scottish, then it will come to mean something to you too.'

As the train pulls into their single platform station from the left Tilly cries triumphantly.

'Towards Glasgow!'

Jumping aboard she sits on the edge of the bench seat, with an ultra-straight back, her hands flat on her knees and a smug look on her face.

However, as they arrive in the big city her confidence fades. Hundreds of people are pouring out onto the platforms, and the air is thick with smoke from the trains, and the cigarettes that all the passengers seem to be dragging on for dear life. Tilly grabs James's hand nervously.

'I can't believe there are so many people here.'

'They're all heading to work. The streets will be quite empty soon.'

'Is this where we're spending our honeymoon?' Tilly looks around anxiously.

'No, but we do have two hours before our connection. Would you like to take a look around the shops, and see if we can find you a new outfit?'

Tilly brightens at the thought, and they head for the station exit.

Tilly has been clutching the bag holding her new dress, ready to jump from the train for the last forty minutes. Finally, the guard shouts *All change please*. They are at the end of the line. Balloch. She's never heard of it. It doesn't look much, but at least they've arrived.

James hoists their suitcase down from the overhead rack and leans out of the window to open the carriage door. Stepping onto the platform ahead of her he turns and offers her his hand. She takes it and once they are on the platform she doesn't let go.

Soon, James is guiding her down Pier Road, odd given that they turned inland from the sea half an hour ago at Dumbarton.

She turns to James and catches the smallest glimpse of a smile at the corners of his mouth and a spark of light in his eye. Anticipation.

They round a corner, and Tilly turns her head to follow James' gaze. Her jaw drops and she gasps. A body of water, too still for a river so probably a lake, stretches away into the distance as far as she can see, but more impressively, behind, and all around, are ridge after ridge of hills and mountains.

'Now do you forgive me for keeping it a secret?' he asks.

She pokes him in the ribs with a smile.

'But where are we? This isn't the sea.'

Isla - 2018

As I flick carefully through the stack of paintings, I see that the majority are images of the shores around Loch Lomond. We took most of our family holidays there. It had been a special place for my parents since their initial honeymoon visit in the early sixties.

I gently open one of the accompanying airmail letters.

Tilly - 1959

Tilly is lying in bed when James enters, carrying a tray, on which he has placed a pot of homemade blackberry jam, tea for two, and a plate of freshly made oatcakes.

She smiles to herself. Her husband is not the best cook, but he takes great pride is his ability to produce oatcakes, porridge, and grilled fish, and rightly so, they are always delicious.

Breakfast in bed is a rare treat, as James is usually up and out early, even if he's not working on the trawler, but today is a special day. It's their first wedding anniversary.

They're back at the loch. This time in a small, rented cottage in Balmaha. It's just a one up, one down, with an outhouse, but they have it all to themselves for four whole days.

Tilly has spent many secret hours on her present for James - which is already safely hidden under her pillow. She's desperate for him to like it.

The first part is practical. Three pairs of thick, hand-knitted socks made from the softest grey wool she could find, to keep his feet warm and cosy inside his boots, whilst he's out on the trawler.

The second part she hopes will be something he can carry with him, at all times. It's a set of large white linen handkerchiefs. She has carefully monogrammed a corner of each with James' initials, entwined with a Scottish thistle for him, and the iris of France for her.

The move to Scotland has been challenging, as she left behind kind people, who were hurt by her decision. Simone and Lorna in particular. But Brittany never felt like home. The community rejected her from the very first day. Then, in the depths of her isolation, along came James.

Cutting herself off from her earlier life and moving here has finally allowed her to leave the anguish behind. To build a new identity and a life that has the possibility of joy and happiness, untouched by the past.

James has provided such unwavering strength and support during this time, and she wants him to understand how grateful she is. For he's seen the many occasions during this last year when she's missed her family intensely. At times she's even gone so far as to have second thoughts.

Without knowing it, James has reassured her every time, with proof of his faithfulness, and commitment to their relationship. His delight at seeing her on his returns from sea is enough to make anyone feel special.

Now, her focus needs to be on preventing anything from happening to him.

James places the tray on the centre of the bed and climbs back in beside her. As he does so he reaches into his bedside table and passes her an envelope.

For a moment she is disappointed. An envelope, after all the trouble she has gone to? At least he has remembered the date.

However, as soon as she opens the envelope, she's flooded with guilt. The outer layer is an invitation to dinner at a restaurant of her choosing, but this is just protection for the next layer. A beautiful watercolour that he must have painted whilst on their honeymoon at Balloch the previous year. Behind this, there is also a thin piece of airmail paper folded carefully in quarters to be the same size as the picture.

She opens it. It is a tribute to her.

Isla - 2018

I'm reluctant to read my father's private thoughts and allow my eye to skim the outpourings of love for his wife, only stopping at the mention of a place, or a name.

Despite this circumspect approach, between the letters and the paintings, I have gained a very vivid picture of my parents' life before I was born, and Da's delight at introducing his new wife, to the Scotland that he loved.

It has been very confusing. I'm experiencing an out-pouring of love and compassion for my parents, and at the same time, I am absolutely furious with them both.

Right now, I can take no more. It's clear that my father knew, all along, that Mam wasn't British. He just forgot to tell me.

A delay of a few days has done nothing to reduce my anger, but I'm travelling tomorrow, and the letters are too numerous, and too precious, to take with me.

The handkerchief itself has an intricate flower design, and the initials J M, hand-stitched with great care by someone. I wonder if it was Mam. She certainly had the skills. I remember her knitting Da new socks for every anniversary, and each year, without fail, he would give her flowers and take her out for a meal.

I always thought that these exchanges were quite mundane and unimaginative, but perhaps they were adjuncts to these other secret and heart-felt exchanges, full of ritual and memory.

There's so much more to my parents' relationship than I ever imagined. It's disconcerting to know that I've been an unwitting third wheel, at many of these special moments between the pair of them. For, whilst they both undoubtedly loved me deeply, that love had nothing on the bond that I'm witnessing here.

If I'm honest, I think that I always felt this. At a deep, unspoken level. There was always something magnetic between the two of them. I could be close to either of them on the outer edge, but I could never occupy the space between them.

The watercolour for their first anniversary is a view of Loch Lomond from the narrow base at Balloch, with the *Maid of the Loch* paddle steamer setting off in all its glory.

The accompanying letter promises that one day they will take a trip on *The Maid*. I wonder if they ever did. Money had always been tight, but Da saved his pennies, and knew how to give us a good time without a lot of expense.

The following year, the view is from further around on the Eastern side of the Loch. The foreground features yellow gorse, and a pathway, that I recognise as the point where the *West Highland Way* leaves Balmaha, for the waterside section, on the way to Fort William.

Tilly - 1960

The small boat docks at the landing stage on Inchcailloch, for James and Tilly to alight. James is deep in conversation with the captain, so Tilly sets off to explore the shore.

A stand of trees is growing right up to the water's edge, and she hurries to take a closer look. Now she feels a fool. Of course, this is freshwater.

She glances over her shoulder. James is still chatting away. Her stomach is rumbling. It's already lunchtime. Their plan is to go straight down the middle of the island, to the beach at Port Bawn for a picnic, leaving the exploring until later.

Knowing how hard it is to stop James talking, once he starts on the subject of boats, she sets off up the path on her own to have a bit of a scout around.

Unfortunately, it isn't long before the path divides. There's still no sign of James, so she collects a few pebbles and sticks and makes an arrow at the junction pointing up the pathway that leads straight ahead.

Hopefully James will see her sign. It will be hard to miss it right here in the middle of the path, but when he's daydreaming, he can be very unaware of his surroundings.

The boat owner mentioned an old burial ground in this direction. Perhaps she will have time to look at it before James catches up with her.

Tilly's stomach growls, bringing her attention back to the moment. She's ravenous and must have been exploring the burial ground a lot longer than she intended.

Where's James? He must have missed the two arrows that she laid for him. She can feel her heart rate rising. She isn't exactly lost. She knows how to find her way back to the landing stage, and she knows how to get to the picnic site. She even knows that there are only three paths on this relatively small island.

Nevertheless, finding James is going to be really difficult. They could walk in circles for hours without catching up with each other.

Tilly retraces her steps to the junction with the central path. Should she return to the landing point? By now he must have started to follow her. She redirects her arrow, pointing it down towards Port Bawn. Then hoists up her skirt and runs down the path as fast as she can.

She needs to catch up with him before he sets off around the perimeter in search of her. Otherwise, there will be no way for her to know which direction he will take.

Isla - 2018

I open the corresponding letter. In it, Da is reminding Mam of a time they spent hours chasing each other around Inchcailloch Island.

I have beautiful childhood memories of that island. A local man provided an ad-hoc ferry service in a small wooden boat that could only hold about ten people. I wonder if he's still operating.

The small number of visitors on each crossing meant that they would quickly disperse, allowing each group a feeling of isolation and adventure. Although, the island itself can't have been much more than a mile long.

Da always chose the hardest route. Taking us up the steep path from the landing stage, in the hope of escaping less adventurous walkers, and of seeing the deer that liked to hide out on the rocky outcrops during the tourist season.

The view from the summit is spectacular. I can recall it in my mind even now. Not only is the vast expanse of the Loch and many of its islands laid out below, but beyond this, the Highlands themselves advance into the distance.

The tip of the island has a beach, and I would always try and persuade Mam to take me directly there without stopping at the graveyard, which I found spooky and sinister.

But Da had a passion for local history and liked to remember the Irish missionary who settled on the island in the eighth century, so I rarely escaped.

As far as I can remember, we never stayed in that cottage in Balmaha as a family, but we stayed at multiple guest-houses in the region, exploring the villages along the shore and occasionally, if things at the shop were going well, and the holiday fund was big enough, Da would hire a small boat for a day or two so that we could explore the further reaches of the Loch.

Those were my favourite times. Mam sitting happily in the bow knitting. Da in his element out on the water, and me learning to manage a tiller, or an outboard motor, under his watchful eye.

In those years, we were truly the ideal happy family. Perhaps that magnetic bond did include me after all.

The remaining images in the bundle are scenes and memories of family holidays around the Loch. Curious to see what the second packet from the dressing table holds, I reach for the parcel that has been so carefully wrapped in tissue paper and tied with a piece of ribbon, probably by my mother.

Tilly - 1964

Tilly is feeling anxious and a little sick. Is the nausea from the anxiety, or the news that she is about to share? She has arranged to meet James on the beach at the entrance to the Seamill Hydro, in the hope that they might go inside afterwards to celebrate. So long as he takes the news the way that she hopes.

She had suspected that she was pregnant for the last few weeks but has only just seen the doctor to have it confirmed. She couldn't have said anything sooner - not until she was sure.

Will she find the words she wants in English?

Perhaps a written note is better.

Isla - 2018

I loosen the ribbon and unwrap the crumpled tissue paper. Inside I find a tiny hand-knitted jumper, suitable for a very young child, and this time a note in my mother's handwriting.

Darling James,
At last, it has happened. You are going to become a father. I know that you will be the best father that any child could ask for, just as you are the best husband.
To the only man I could ever love, for the moment when our child arrives.
Yours ever,
Tilly.

    I can barely breathe. The lump in my throat is so big, and the tears are falling silently onto the wool of the jumper as it lies in my lap. I quickly shake them off before they can sink in and do any damage.

James - 1964

James looks from the tiny parcel in his lap, to his beautiful wife. They are going to have a child! He can see what this means to her.

When they first met, her wish for a family of her own had been one of the things they had discussed, in hushed undertones, as she pretended to read at his bedside. Then later, when he returned, and she agreed to marry him, talk of that future included him too. Now, at last, with a child on the way, their dream is complete.

Da! ... Someone is going to call him Da! ... He can feel a burning energy in the centre of his chest, and a warmth spreading upward and outward to his fingertips. He wants to leap up, and run down onto the sand, turning cartwheels as he goes.

Instead, as his smile spreads, he reaches out to Tilly, kissing her with every ounce of the passion that he feels. Despite the other visitors to the beach. He draws her up onto his knee and rocks her backwards and forwards shouting, 'We're having a baby!'

Thirteen

Isla - 2018

I've been to Paris many times, but never with these eyes. I'm keen to find the city of my mother's birth and to get a feel for the area in which her parents lived. I wonder how much choice they had in that.

To our twenty-first century eyes, city centres are prime-real estate, but during the 1930s, when my grandparents were living in the tenth arrondissement, the two major rail terminals in the area would have brought hundreds of coal-fired trains.

The air would have been thick with the heavy particulates of coal and wood smoke. A very different experience to the invisible pollution that I accept as a city-dweller in Dortmund.

An address in this area, at that time, suggests that my grandparents were not wealthy. Those with a little money who remained in the area would have headed upwards, out of the pollution, to the top of tall apartment buildings. Without an actual address, I can't tell whether this was a possibility for my family.

If they'd been middle class, they would have been more likely to take advantage of the newly expanded metro system and escape to the growing suburbs.

I take my first breath above ground as I exit the station and get a quick reminder that the air in Paris is still far from clean.

The streets are full of people from all over the world. I'm certain that many, like me, are tourists in transit, as every third person seems to be pulling a suitcase.

The area around the Gare du Nord is a real mixture of old and new. There are run-down and almost derelict buildings that would certainly have been here in my grandparents' time. Some have been lovingly restored or cleaned up by the companies that own them but sandwiched in between are a smattering of brand-new developments.

I've always loved the way that old French buildings have massive, metal gates onto the street that guard the entrances to secret courtyards. Somewhere, behind one of these, my grandparents would have gained access to their apartment.

By early afternoon I am in my hire car on the A6 heading towards Barantan. It's a small village on the outskirts of Vichy. I'm not in a hurry and technically this is the most direct route. The two lanes in each direction are plenty for the quantity of traffic, and there are enough bends in the road for me to stay alert. From time-to-time, tree-lined verges give way to open fields, or industrial ribbon development, but in essence, the landscape is wide and flat. I can't wait to reach the Auvergne. I have heard so much about its mountains and forests.

Towards Les Andrivaux the ground becomes more undulating, and as I approach Les Gadons, the road is lined with white, red roofed, two-storey houses. I become hopeful that this is the start of the beautiful scenery.

However, as I drive through Champcourt the area takes on an industrial feel, with the buildings constructed in the latter half of the twentieth century. So, I'm relieved to find that Vichy itself has a real flavour of Paris. Many old buildings are three-storeys or more, with wrought iron balconies and grand frontages.

Barantan therefore comes as a huge disappointment. Not only are there no mountains, but the incredibly flat farmland was obviously ideal for post-war building. I am surrounded by bungalows and two storey new builds.

I've been here twenty minutes and driven along every street and dirt track in the area. I had been counting on there being a Mairie for public records, or a church with gravestones. It seems that Barantan is not big enough for either.

Utterly dejected, I park up on the side of the road, and take out my phone. The nearest Mairie is in Le Vernet, a few kilometres away. It's worth a try. They may hold records for this village too.

I push open the door and try to muster up my best French. I've continued to practice since Mam died, especially in the weeks since I made my decision to come to France, but my questions are complex and soon I'm stumbling.

'English?' suggests the middle-aged woman behind the counter.

'Yes please!' I reply, hugely relieved.

'I'm trying to find out about some people who lived in this area, who might have been my relatives.'

The woman's eyes light up.

'I love this sort of thing. Do you have an address, or just their names?'

'I have their death certificates, and I know they came from Barantan.' I pass the documents over.

'Excellent. I'm sure we'll be able to tell you something. Let me see. Oh, this one says the death was registered by *Rory Stewart of Barantan*. I know about him.'

'You do? Who is he?' I'm so excited I can hardly breathe. 'I thought he sounded Scottish, but I guess that's not likely.'

'No, you're right, he was. His daughter taught me at school when I was little. She liked telling us her father's story. He came to France to fight, during the First World War, but fell in love with a local woman, her mother Dominique, so he stayed. It was such a romantic story. I never forgot it.'

I wonder if he knew my father's family. Perhaps that's how my parents met.

'That's beautiful,' I agree, 'but it doesn't help me work out who Chloe and Joseph are.'

'Oh, but it will, because Lorna Stewart is still alive. She lives here in Le Vernet. I often see her when she's doing her shopping. I'm sure she would speak to you. She doesn't have any family, and she likes a chat.'

I can feel a lump forming in my throat. An actual person to talk to. This is incredible.

The woman glances at her watch.

'Can you meet me at the bar down the road after work? I'll try and contact her to see if she can join us there.'

'Thank you so much!' I say, extending my hand. 'My name's Isla by the way.'

'Lis,' she says, grasping my hand. 'Pleased to meet you. This is so exciting!'

Fourteen

Isla – 2018

Lis and I are drinking white wine at a table just inside the bar when an elderly lady with curly, iron-grey hair enters. Despite the curvature of her spine, and her use of a walking stick, she makes a beeline for our table, walking briskly, with a firm stride.

She bends her knees slightly as she approaches, so that she can look directly into my eyes. Then, with a huge smile on her face, she stretches her free arm towards me and in perfect English, with a warm, rich, Scottish accent, says,

'You're Clothilde's daughter.'

I nearly fall off my seat with shock, and tears spring from my eyes.

I lean on the table for support as she crosses the remaining distance between us and puts her arm around my shoulders.

'It is so lovely to meet you Isla. I've waited fifty-four years for this moment. But I guess this must mean that darling Clothilde is dead.'

She hugs me tight as I weep onto her bosom.

For the first time since the funerals, I am with someone who loved Mam as much as I did, and she knows who I am. No complex explanations needed.

In a few well-chosen words, she has also let me know that she understands the complexity of loving my mother.

When my tears subside, Lis reaches across and hands me a tissue. Then rising, she pulls out a chair, and helps Lorna to settle comfortably.

'This is incredible. You actually know who Isla is!' Lis turns towards me shaking her head in disbelief. 'I didn't mention your name when I called. I just said that someone was looking for information about Rory Stewart.'

Puzzled, I'm desperate to ask how Lorna knows who I am, but I'm still too shocked to speak.

Lorna smiles indulgently at me.

'You look very like her, and you still look like your baby picture. Your mother's last communication with me was to send me a photograph of the two of you together, not long after you were born. I have looked at that photograph so often over the years. I couldn't help but recognise you.'

'That's so sweet, but I'm a little confused.' Lis confesses. 'Who's Clothilde? The names Isla gave me were Chloe and Joseph.'

'Clothilde was my mother's name when she lived in France, although, I always knew her as Tilly.' I explain. 'Camille was her mother. I'm hoping Lorna can help with where Chloe and Joseph fit in.' I add, having finally found the ability to speak.

'Isla's mother and I were best friends from the moment that she arrived here. She was a very grown up four-year-old. I was a bit older. There were hardly any children in our village, so we became inseparable.'

For a moment Lorna develops a faraway look in her eyes. Her face softens. Lis and I can see that she's grappling with powerful emotions, so we wait patiently until she's ready to continue.

'Clothilde and her mother arrived in 1940. Refugees from Paris. Henri - your grandfather - worked for the railways. The plan had been for the family to escape to Brittany, where his own family lived. I don't know if he intended for them to flee the country by boat, or to stay there. Tragically, just before they were due to leave, Henri was killed in a bombing raid on a transport depot.'

'Oh my god, how awful!' I can't prevent myself interrupting.

Lorna nods sadly in acknowledgment but carries on.

'Camille didn't want to live with people she barely knew, so instead, she swapped her tickets and brought Clothilde here, to the Auvergne.'

'Poor woman! I can't imagine how she held it together.' Lis exclaims. 'Newly widowed with a tiny child.'

'No one knew she was coming.' Lorna says with regret. 'The train arrived very late and the two of them ended up sleeping overnight in the parklands beside the river Allier.'

'Mam must have been terrified.'

I can't really remember anything from when I was four, but my life at that time was calm and ordinary.

'Do you think a four-year-old could create lasting memories of an ordeal like that?'

'I know for sure that she did,' Lorna is emphatic. 'We shared a bed many times over the years, and she had a recurring nightmare based on that day. I was often woken by her fearful and erratic breathing. She would writhe in the bed, but the most distressing thing was that she would never call out. The need to keep quiet had been so deeply impressed upon her, that she was silent even in her sleep.'

My eyes fill with tears as I remember Mam thrashing around in her bed at Suncrest with her fist jammed into her mouth to muffle her cries of distress.

I don't want to cry in public, so speaking brightly, I change the subject.

'So, this makes Chloe and Joseph Mam's grandparents.'

I'm glad to have finally got everyone sorted. They're *my* great-grandparents. I'm relieved that Mam and Camille had loving people to take them in after the shock of Henri's death.

'Were they kind?' I look hopefully at Lorna, 'I can't imagine losing my Da when I was just a wee mite.'

I turn to include Lis in my explanation.

'My father also died a little while ago. As a fully grown woman I'm finding it hard enough to cope with the loss. As a little child you're so dependent on your parents! I can't imagine it. Perhaps people were tougher in war time?'

Lorna doesn't react to my last remark but carries on with her tale.

'Chloe and Joseph were lovely warm folk, but they were not people of the world. They had both grown up in this area and farmed the land all their lives. They had fallen out with Camille because she'd made the decision to move to Paris in 1929, in search of adventure. They just couldn't understand why someone would make such a choice. They'd been even worse about her decision to marry Henri, so bringing their young child back here was a difficult step for Camille.'

I think of my own decision to leave a small community in search of greater challenges and new experiences. It sounds as if my grandmother and I might have had a lot in common. Could this have been another reason why Mam found it difficult to deal with my teenage aspirations. Did I remind her of her mother in a way that was painful?

'I think history repeated itself. Mam and I didn't see eye to eye when I left our village in Scotland on a move to Germany's industrial heartland. It took us a long time to heal the rift.'

Lorna nods in commiseration. She really does understand what my mother was like.

'Camille was a real fish out of water when she arrived in Barantan. I'll never forget it. She was wearing an elegantly cut suit and a ridiculous pair of satin gloves. No one on the farms had ever seen such things, let alone worn them. Hands were always needed for one mucky job or another.'

I can just imagine her arrival.

'The only concession that she had made to her surroundings was that she'd swapped her favoured heels for a pair of brogues. Joseph found it very difficult to accept her back.'

'Oh, Poor Camille.' Lis interjects.

I'm startled. I've been so engrossed in what Lorna has been saying, that I'd forgotten Lis' presence. A part of me wishes that she wasn't here. These memories feel special and private, but the truth is, I would have left the area without knowing any of this if it wasn't for her assistance.

I'm therefore relieved when Lis says,

'Unfortunately, I must return home to cook dinner for my family. Thank you for a most interesting day.'

We say our farewells, and Lorna and I are left staring at each other across the table.

'I really can't believe that you're here in France.'

Lorna reaches for my hand.

'Tell me, do you have family? Are they here with you?'

'No, no it's just me.'

I expect to see the usual disappointment at my answer, but to the contrary Lorna moves excitedly on to her next question.

'So, what do you do?'

'Well, officially I'm European Manager for a company dealing with specialist micro-systems technology. They're based in the North Rhine Westphalia, so I live in Dortmund.'

Lorna looks puzzled but not defeated.

'What are micro systems?'

'We deal with technological developments and their applications for any product the size of a micrometre, that's one millionth of a metre.'

'That's impossible. How on earth can people make anything so small?' Lorna looks baffled.

'Well, that's just it, people can't, but machines can. The parts are used across a huge range of industries.'

'Such as?'

Lorna is now genuinely interested, which is lovely for me. Most people glaze over when I start talking about work. It's one of the reasons I find chit-chat so difficult. People always ask what I do, and then hurriedly make an excuse to move away when they don't know how to respond. With joy, I take this rare opportunity to elaborate.

'Well, micro-systems technology is essential in the motor industry, communications and electronics manufacturing, and there are even medical and pharmaceutical applications.'

'How astonishing! I feel feeble just thinking of all these tiny, tiny products keeping our world running. You're obviously a very bright woman like your grandmother.'

'Camille?'

'Yes. According to my mother, one of the main reasons that Camille left Barantan for Paris was that she had a phenomenal brain. It had never been stretched by the local school, and Camille was impatient to see the world and to challenge herself.'

'I wonder if Mam knew that.' I ponder out loud. 'She never mentioned that I took after her mother. Oh, not that I would say I have a phenomenal brain.' I flush with embarrassment. 'Just that I was very interested in school.'

'The greatest tragedy of Clothilde's life, was that she was denied time with her parents.'

'Both of them?' I ask. 'I know that you said Henri was killed.'

My mind turns to the child evacuees of Britain. I guess children who grew up in wartime were often separated from their parents, although I'm not aware of such a thing in France.

I look up in the hope that she will explain, but find that she is bent double, reaching for a scarf that has dropped to the floor. She hasn't heard my question.

As Lorna sits back up, she's already speaking, and her mind has obviously gone in another direction.

'Your mother wrote to me only twice after she married your father. The first time, to say that she was beginning a new life, and much as she loved me, she had to start afresh, and would not be in contact again. The second time, she broke her own rule, to send me that photograph of you. It came with a short message that you had been born, the two of you were well, and she hoped that I too knew the joy of having a child of my own.'

I can see the sadness of Lorna's childless life cross her face. At the same time, I feel an intense warmth spread through the front of my body. Mam had truly loved me.

'I can see how much you cared for Mam.' I say, reaching out to rest my hand on Lorna's arm. 'You must have been devastated when she cut herself off.'

'It's one of the deepest sorrows of my life.' Lorna admits. 'As the years went by, I came to understand … she was a very disturbed young woman. If compartmentalising her mind, and cutting off from her past, brought her peace, from the recurring nightmares and all the trauma, then, in my opinion, it was a price that needed to be paid. I felt her loss, but she deserved happiness, and it was clear that she had found that with James.'

Clothilde - 1940

Maman hurried Clothilde out of the apartment this morning without plaiting her hair, because they have a train to catch. As a result, Clothilde is repeatedly shaking her head, to rid herself of the blonde curtain, that keeps falling across her face as they scurry along the pavement.

The streets of Paris are packed with people running and shouting. There are car horns blaring, and everywhere she looks, people are loading odd things that should be in their houses - like paintings, blankets, and pots and pans - onto carts.

Clothilde knows the way to the train station. They come here often with Papa. He hasn't been at home for the last few nights, and she is looking forward to seeing him.

The station is much busier than usual, and they have to stand in a long queue at the ticket window.

Maman looks anxious. There is something going on. There are so many more people here than usual. Clothilde looks around for Papa. For a moment she thinks she sees him, but then the man turns around and he has a moustache. That's definitely not Papa.

It's Maman's turn at the window. She's trying to change some tickets. Clothilde doesn't understand. Her arm is getting tired, so she puts her small suitcase flat on the ground and sits down on it.

It has her nightdress, her teddy bear, a jumper and scarf, a few skirts and tops, and some underwear. At the last minute she had added the storybook from her bedside table. It didn't really fit. The catch on the suitcase had only just closed when she sat on it. Now she's worried that the whole thing will pop open and spill all her belongings onto the platform as they board the train.

Maman is finished. She has the new tickets between her teeth, and their big suitcases in her hands. She nods with her head towards the platforms, with such a pleading look in her sad eyes that Clothilde knows she must hurry, and not get lost.

The train is not what she expects. There are no carriages with comfortable seats like the ones they have been on before. These are like carts. They are smelly and very high up. Maman lifts her up with the baggage, and then wriggles up beside her.

More and more people are coming. Clothilde is scared. Surely there is no more room. Maman has made a pile with their bags and is standing up against it holding Clothilde tightly as she sits on top.

Clothilde tries to ask about Papa, but Maman doesn't answer. She just places her hand over Clothilde's mouth, and looking deep into her eyes, shakes her head.

It has been a long day. Clothilde slept for part of the journey, leaning up against Maman as she sat on top of the cases. However, the sleep doesn't seem to have made her less tired. The grown-ups are frightened. She can feel it in the air.

She has never been with so many people, squashed up into such a tight space before. It smells awful. It's not just the smelliness of the carriage. Their human sweat really stinks. It's not the normal smell of sweat, like Papa when he first comes home from work.

She can hear a woman crying, and two men are trying to fight each other, although they have no room to move their arms.

Camille and Clothilde prepare to leave the train, along with all the other people. The station starts with the letter V, but Clothilde can't read the rest.

'Time to get off now, don't let go of my coat.'

This is the first thing Maman has said to her since they climbed into the train in Paris. During the journey she had hugged Clothilde a lot, but she hadn't replied to any of her questions. Instead, she had repeatedly placed her hand over her mouth and kissed the top of her head, before resuming her embrace.

Clothilde is really frightened. Something is badly wrong, but she doesn't know what. Papa should be here. They had all talked about going on a long train journey together to see his sisters. She's looking forward to meeting her aunts. Papa says they have been waiting more than four years to meet her and will want to play with her every day. She can't remember their names, but she knows that they live by the sea. She's never been to the seaside, but she has seen pictures.

Clothilde's arm is growing tired, but Maman is already carrying the big cases so can't take hers, and she dare not let go of Maman's coat to swap hands, as there are so many people here pushing and shoving.

The locals are sitting on their doorsteps, watching all the passengers from the train trudge by. They are dressed differently from the people arriving from Paris and they are not being very friendly. They don't smile, they just stare as the people pass by along their streets.

It's dark already, and the streets are now littered with people sitting on their luggage, with blank expressions on their faces. Clothilde is unsure where she and her mother are going, and it seems that Maman doesn't know either, as she keeps walking up to buildings and ringing the bell, only to be greeted by someone shaking their heads. Maman then turns around, and they resume walking.

At the next building they try Maman seems more hopeful, as there is a sign in the window. There are big gates, and a small courtyard. Clothilde likes this place. The two-storey building has three little houses like dog kennels on the roof, each with its own tiny window.

The door in the centre of the house opens as Maman approaches, and a woman carrying a dishcloth starts to speak. At the same time a man steps out on to the balcony above and starts gesturing angrily at them to leave.

Maman hurries back down the front steps, and rejoins Clothilde, who has been waiting just inside the gate. She shakes her head, picks up the bags and hurries back out into the street.

Maman turns around and leads them off in a different direction. The buildings end. There are trees, and grass, and an inky blackness ahead of them that might be water.

Maman puts the bags down under a tree. Off to each side Clothilde can see indistinct shapes in the dark and hear muttering voices. She clutches Maman's hand tightly and starts to shake. There are two green eyes in that bush. Is it a monster waiting to pull them into the water when their backs are turned?

There are people here too. Perhaps they will protect her from the monster. She can hear arguing and an occasional baby crying. Many of the voices sound like big children. It's scary without any lights and its cold. There is a strong wind running along the water. Now that her eyes are used to the dark it looks like a river.

Maman opens one of the cases and pulls out her green lamb's wool dress.

'Clothilde, put this on over your clothes. It will keep you warm. I know how much you love it.'

Clothilde does indeed love to stroke it whenever Maman wears it.

Maman then spreads another cotton dress on the ground and creates walls around it with the baggage. Maman sits down on the dress with her back against the tree and beckons Clothilde - now swamped in the oversized dress - to lie beside her.

As Clothilde lies down, with her head in her mother's lap, Maman spreads her overcoat across the pair of them.

'Sleep now ma chérie, we will stay here until morning.'

Isla - 2018

Lorna is sitting incredibly still, her mind turned inwards as she shares my mother's story.

'Their flight from Paris was only part of it. There was some kind of incident in the area by the river where they slept the night. I didn't ever hear the details, but I overheard Camille talking to Chloe, and she mentioned a stabbing, with lots of screaming in the middle of the night. She and Clothilde had to hide in the bushes until it was over. They weren't able to go far in the dark, but as soon as dawn broke, they packed up and slipped away.'

Clothilde - 1940

Clothilde wakes to find her nose being pressed into her mother's shoulder. It's making it hard to breathe, and Maman's arms are holding her tightly. It's usually Papa that carries her to bed. She lifts her head to look around and Maman's hand comes down fast over her mouth and nose.

Terrified, she kicks herself straight, and the two of them fall to the ground, but Maman doesn't let go. Now, she is lying on top of her as she brings her mouth to Clothilde's ear.

'Shh! Be quiet. There is a bad man. Be still.'

Clothilde does as she is told.

'Hurry! Under that bush. Hide!'

Maman points to where the monster lives.

Clothilde wriggles and shakes her head vehemently.

Maman points again urging her forward, but Clothilde is terrified of the monster, she flings herself into her mother's chest crying silently.

At the same moment a hideous scream breaks the quiet night air, and Maman dives under the bush taking Clothilde with her. Now Clothilde understands. However, frightened she is of the monster, Maman is more frightened of the man.

Clothilde can feel a gentle nudging on her arm. It is just annoying enough to wake her. She opens her eyelids and looks straight up into Maman's face. Her eyes look strange. This is not the warm smiling morning face that Clothilde is used to. Maman looks as if she's been awake all night. She has her finger on her lips. Clothilde understands that she mustn't speak.

As sleep finally leaves her, she remembers that they're not at home. She rolls her head to take in her surroundings. To her surprise there are thousands of other people scattered across the parkland all around them. They have all slept the night here beside what she now sees is a wide river.

Turning her head to her left she spots the bush under which they hid last night. The man with the knife! Where is the man with the knife?

Clothilde sits bolt upright, her heart racing at the thought, but Maman is ready. She rests one hand on Clothilde's shoulder, and strokes her hair with the other, to reassure her. There's no sign of him now.

Repeating her gesture to be quiet Maman shows that they must pack up. Most other people are still asleep. From the way that she is glancing around it doesn't look like Maman trusts them.

Maman is hurrying ahead of Clothilde along the water's edge. Occasionally she glances back to check that she is being followed. There are so many new things to look at, Clothilde is finding it difficult to walk quickly.

On the outskirts of town Maman suddenly pulls Clothilde to one side in the shelter of a doorway. A string of soldiers on horseback ride past, the sound of their horses' hooves ringing out clearly in the early morning silence.

What is happening and where is Papa?

Fifteen

Isla - 2018

The morning is warm, and I have the air-conditioning going full blast in the car so that Lorna and I can travel in comfort. Having talked for ages last night about the last fifty years of my life, we are now heading to Barantan so that I can hear more about Mam's life before I was born.

We reach a five-way junction, and my satnav is telling me to turn right, but Lorna places a steadying hand on my arm.

'Can we make a detour Isla? I want to show you the route your mother took the day she arrived in Barantan. We will obviously be going in the opposite direction, but I want you to imagine a little four-year-old, carrying her own small suitcase, whilst her mother struggled with the two huge bags, rammed with every possession she thought she might need to support them for the rest of their lives.'

I look across at her. Somehow her words have more impact now that we are out on this road.

Clothilde - 1940

The pace of their walking has slowed considerably, as Maman's bags are heavy, and she keeps putting them down for a rest. Every time she does this Clothilde takes the chance to sit on her own case and rub her sore hand and arm. Thankfully, now that they are away from the crowds, she no longer has to hold on to Maman's coat, and can swap hands as often as she likes.

They have reached a big crossroads with fields on all sides. To the left she can see a cluster of houses with a hill rising in the distance. To the right the path slopes slightly upwards towards the sky, and ahead, the way that they are going, the path sweeps around a small cluster of trees and then disappears down over the brow of the hill.

They have been walking, for what feels like hours, and Clothilde is hungry. Maman has promised her a biscuit for breakfast once they reach the cluster of houses on the horizon.

Clothilde has never been to the countryside before. It's a bit like when she goes to the park in Paris, but there are less flowers and more green plants. Clothilde is glad that this bit of road is very flat. It is easier to walk. Carrying this suitcase up hill is hard.

There is the sound of an engine travelling fast towards them, and Maman pulls Clothilde into a thicket to hide behind a large, ivy-covered log. Clothilde knows better than to speak. Nothing is clear. Maman seems to want to hide from everybody. She only relaxes a little bit when there is no one else around.

A moment later, a large motorbike races past them. The rider is wearing a helmet and goggles and has a very determined set to his mouth. Maman stays where she is, listening for a while, before helping Clothilde to climb back out onto the road, so that they can resume their journey.

Isla - 2018

The satnav says we are on Rue des Michalets. It's a long, narrow road curving across wide flat open farmland. Even now there are only a smattering of buildings along the way. We gain enough elevation to see Vichy spread out before us in the distance, but at the junction with the Rue de la Jonchère we are forced to stop as the route turns into a private road.

I pull over and sit holding onto the steering wheel. It is probably only four kilometres into Vichy, but the thought of walking such a long way, with a tiny child, exhausted after a frightening night sleeping rough in a park, is awful. To do so, whilst also carrying two giant suitcases is unimaginable.

I remember the day that I tried to walk home from the DIY store carrying two five-litre cans of paint. I thought my arms were going to drop off after the first fifteen minutes, and although I travel with suitcases all the time for work, they're rarely large, and always have wheels.

Camille's bags would have been made of heavy leather. I have no idea how she managed.

I turn the car around and we retrace our route, eventually taking the turning into Barantan. Lorna asks me to pull up in the shade of a small copse.

'This was my parents farm.'

I am looking at a small collection of modern houses with hard surface parking and back gardens consisting of about fifty square metres of mown lawns.

'It's hard to imagine.'

'It was home, but I understood that we couldn't stay. The land was never capable of high yields, and as farming methods changed it was uneconomical to continue.'

I look across and see sadness on her face.

'That must have been hard.'

'Selling the land was the right choice. I had decided to become a teacher, and I had no siblings to take over from my parents. But it almost broke them to move to Le Vernet.'

'I can imagine.' I say, nodding gently, as I cast my eyes across this soulless collection of bungalows. 'So, what about Mam, where did she live? You said you were neighbours.'

Lorna extends her arm and points through the windscreen ahead of us.

'The land on the left-hand side of the road, between here and the junction, all belonged to your great-grandfather. The farmhouse and courtyard of out-buildings were on the corner.'

I can't believe it. Not a trace of the farm is left. I'm not sure what I had hoped for from this visit with Lorna, particularly as I came here yesterday and scoured the area with no success, but the disappointment is bitter.

Lorna rests her hand sympathetically on my knee.

'The physical reminders may be gone, but I can still tell you a lot about their lives.'

I turn to her as she continues.

'It's their stories that will help you understand who they were.'

I give a nod and a shrug.

'For example, during the war none of the farms had horses because they were all taken for the war effort, so all the heavy work was done by the cattle. Every now and then they would be taken to the blacksmith at the top of the village to be shod. Joseph's animals really didn't like it.'

I'm puzzled.

'Weren't there tractors in 1940?'

'Our farms had never generated enough profit for expensive farm machinery. Joseph's animals were a bit of a liability. I've got the scar to prove it!'

Lorna points to a small, jagged scar just below her left cheekbone.

'What happened?' I ask, eager to be drawn back in time.

'One of the young oxen kicked the farrier, slipped his rope and made a dash for home.'

Clothilde - 1941

Clothilde and Lorna are playing hopscotch in the lane. The grid is marked out with twigs, and it is Clothilde's turn. She is taking aim with her stone when Lorna suddenly shouts.

'Look out!' and pushes her hard towards the verge.

Clothilde falls to the ground and is furious, until four huge hooves thunder past within inches of her face.

She turns to see Lorna who is dabbing a bloody scratch on her cheek.

'Are you ok?' Clothilde asks in concern.

'I'm fine, it didn't get me. It was one of our twigs. It struck me as it flew up in the air. I'm ok.'

Clothilde looks down at the lane. Three squashed and broken twigs are all that remains of their grid. They are so lucky to have escaped being trampled.

Away in the distance she can see a group of adults from neighbouring farms waving their arms and trying to direct the animal into a field.

Isla - 2018

'It really wasn't the creature's fault.' Lorna continues. 'The cattle had never been intended as working animals, and Joseph had enormous difficulty trying to train them to pull the plough and do all the other work that the horses had done previously.'

'We forget how much harder wartime farming must have been without fuel for machinery, and with many of the animals taken as well. But at least you must have eaten well, unlike people in the cities.'

'Not really, we were very closely watched, to be sure that the food we produced went to the soldiers, and to the urban areas that weren't producing for themselves. I remember we ate a lot of soup made from salvaged corners of damaged or infested vegetables.'

My stomach turns at the thought.

Clothilde - 1941

The kitchen is filled with the strange smell of the roasted soya beans, that the adults are grinding, and drinking in place of coffee. Clothilde is waiting patiently for the spoonful of her vitamin supplement. It's a special treat. Only the children get this ration and it's deliciously sweet.

She and Lorna have been secretly scrounging wild figs and blackberries from the hedgerows, but that's finished now. It will be months before the peaches and other fruit trees are once again able to provide sweetness to mealtimes at the farm.

This is not the only change that's happened in their household this winter. Proper meals have been replaced with soups and other single pot creations. Her grandparents and the two single farm labourers are working too hard to sit around a table all together.

Instead, the pot is on the stove, ready for any hungry person to help themselves when they come in from the cold.

In some ways this is easier for them all because absences are less notable, but it makes it hard for Clothilde to feel part of a family. In recent weeks she's only returned to the farmhouse to sleep, not that anyone seems to notice.

Lorna's home is different. She and her parents spend hours talking together in their kitchen. Her parents are just as busy. Dominique is usually doing some form of meal preparation or mending, and Rory is always tinkering with something, yet they still manage to create a feeling of homeliness and welcome.

Isla - 2018

My eyes are open, but not seeing, as Lorna continues.

'We did have the possibility of catching rabbits to improve on the soup. My father would take me out at dawn and dusk with the shotgun. He wouldn't let Clothilde come, because he thought she was too little and would make too much noise. I, on the other hand, was in training, so that I could go out on my own after the rabbits.'

'But you can't have been much more than six yourself. Were you even big enough to hold a shotgun?'

'You're right. I was seven years old when my father first took me out. I was quite tall for my age, but I admit, I was scared of the gun, and I liked the rabbits. I didn't want to shoot them. But I was also very hungry.'

I think of my own, comfortable life in West Kilbride at the age of seven. Mam preparing family meals in the kitchen, with an endless supply of unsold fish from the shop. Building sandcastles on the beach or walking in the hills with Da, every Sunday, because he had the day off. I can see that Mam and Lorna had been largely unsupervised as children and been forced to grow up much faster than me.

We drive a little further along the road and pull into a gateway where a field slopes down to a stream.

'Your Mam and I would spend hours here with fishing rods made out of sticks and string, hoping to catch fish, but I don't remember us ever having any luck. I think it is quite likely that the stream was dead, we certainly weren't allowed to drink from it.'

I can't imagine Mam fishing, she always left that to Da. Apart from walking and the occasion swim - although she hated cold water - she always seemed to enjoy more indoor pursuits, like knitting and sewing.

'Fresh water was actually quite a problem here. We had to collect it from the well. But before we did, we had to lift out the milk and the cheese which were stored there in a bucket to keep them cool.'

'So, no refrigerators?'

'No. No electricity, and no running water inside either. About once every couple of weeks my mother would send us to the well for ten pails of water. She would boil six of them in a giant vat on the stove, and they would be poured, along with some cold water, into the bathtub that sat in the middle of the kitchen.

Clothilde and I, by this point, would be deeply grey with dirt. We would be scrubbed all over with carbolic soap to be sure we hadn't picked up any lice, and then sent away whilst my parents took their turns.'

Clothilde - 1941

Winter has been harsh. It's not quite as cold as last year, but as the war goes on supplies of every kind run lower and lower. There is no spare fuel, so the kitchen is the only warm room in the house. Clothilde has learnt to volunteer for all tasks that involve caring for the animals, however smelly they may be.

It's hard physical work, and right now her blood is pumping as she mucks out the stall. But somehow the blood never seems to reach her extremities. Here with the animals, there is usually a moment between chores when she can rest her painful hands against the warmth of the animals' bodies. Unlike when she tends the vegetable patch when her icy fingertips turn blue despite her exertion.

The cattle are the best, as their huge bodies generate a lot of heat, and their hair is soft as she runs her fingers the wrong way against their coats. The feathers of the chickens make them colder to touch, but if you pick them up and cuddle them for a moment the warmth comes through.

The shaggy coat of the billy goat is lovely and warm, and looks perfect for nestling your hands in, but it's hard to get close to his body, as his horns are dangerous, and he's quite grumpy. However, the females are pregnant, so hopefully there will be little kids to play with soon.

Lorna's papa says that the soldiers in the last war used to bathe their hands in urine when they had chilblains like this. He says doing this, and then wearing mittens, is the answer. But it sounds disgusting, and chores are hard to do with mittens on.

Isla - 2018

I look across at Lorna sitting next to me in the car.

'You speak as if Mam lived with you,' I say, puzzled, 'but she had her own family here.'

'There's something I haven't told you yet.' I see Lorna hesitate. 'Although your mother came here with Camille, they didn't have much time together.'

"Why not?'

I can't bear this. Poor Mam. What can have happened? She must have needed her mother so badly.

'All adults had to contribute during war time, and Camille's secretarial and translating experience in Paris meant that she was sent to work in the government offices in Vichy. Meanwhile, Clothilde remained here with Joseph and Chloe.'

'So, Mam lost her father, and then almost immediately was separated from her mother and left with what to her were total strangers?'

'Yes. It was a desperate time in her life. Clothilde was completely confused when she got here. She had been prepared for a relocation to be with her Marec relatives in Brittany. Then the plan changed overnight, and she had no advance warning about the farm, or her maternal grandparents. Camille hadn't even told her of Henri's death until she got here, as she couldn't face making the journey with a grieving child.'

Lorna is pulling at her own fingernails in response to the memory.

'Clothilde's ability to trust was completely shattered.'

Clothilde - 1940

Clothilde is mystified. Despite what Papa told her, there is no sign of the sea, nor of her aunts. Instead, these people they spent last night with are her mother's parents.

Yesterday they walked for hours, and all she saw was fields. Papa had said that the train station was close to the beach, and yet where they camped in the park definitely wasn't a beach, and the water wasn't the sea!

Maman has brought her outside to feed the chickens and see if they have laid any eggs, but she seems worried, and they haven't started either task. Maman is just staring at the chickens as they walk around.

'Why are we here?' Clothilde asks, hoping that this time she might get a reply. Normally Maman chats away, showing her new things, asking her what she can see, reading her stories, saying hello to everyone they meet.

In the last two days, the only brief times she heard her mother's voice were in the parkland, and on the long walk here, when she told fairytales and fables to help stop Clothilde from crying.

Maman has spoken in whispers to the adults since they arrived, and Clothilde is very frightened that something is seriously wrong.

'Where's Papa?' she tries again. 'I thought we were going to the seaside.'

As her mother is still not speaking, Clothilde takes her hand in the hope of leading her on an egg hunt, but instead Camille squats down beside her and takes her other hand as well. Looking deep into her daughter's eyes she says.

'Clothilde, I have some terrible news for you. Papa won't be joining us. He is dead. He was killed at the railyard by a German bomb. I didn't tell you in Paris because I wanted us to get here first, to your grandparents who will help keep you safe.'

'Papa's not coming? What about swimming in the sea together?'

All Clothilde knows is Papa is not coming. No cuddles, no stories at bedtime.

Camille stops speaking, unable to continue. Tears are pouring down her face. Clothilde sees her mother's tears and her bottom lip starts to tremble. Her face crumples, and she starts to cry.

'They've hurt Papa?'

Clothilde pulls her hands free from her mother's grip and starts beating her fists against her mother's chest, staring up into her face, pleading for her to say that this isn't true. She becomes hysterical when her mother's next words are.

'Darling, Papa is dead.'

Isla - 2018

Lorna opens the car window to let in a little air.

'Although Camille was in Vichy most of the time, during the summer months, with the longer daylight hours, she could walk back here after work, see Clothilde for an hour or so, and still return to Vichy before dark. In winter she was restricted to visiting just once a week on her day off.'

I think of my journey here which had brought me through Vichy. It's a short enough drive, but exhausting, on foot, after a tiring day at work. I hope that Camille's determination to see Mam would have given her added strength.

'I think that the enforced separation from her mother was why Clothilde preferred to be with me whenever possible. I became like an elder sister.'

'You know, that's what it feels like. I feel like you're my aunt. The way that you talk about Mam, and the warmth, it feels like family.'

I can feel myself blushing. This openness isn't my way. I've never been one to speak about emotion, not even to my own parents, but the immediate connection I felt with Lorna was so striking. I'm worried that if I don't say anything she may be gone from my life in a day or two when I leave the area.

'Perhaps it's also our shared Scottish heritage.' Lorna suggests. 'The French find me very different, despite the fact that I've spent my whole life here, and my mother was a Frenchwoman through and through.'

I feel a broad smile stretching across my face.

'So, your father had a big influence on your outlook, as well as on your accent and your bilingualism?'

'Oh yes, I was a real Daddy's girl. But it wasn't just that. Clothilde and I unexpectedly spent a lot of time with him during the spring of 1941. He had an accident and broke his leg. It was a disaster for our farm, as that only left my mother to do all the hard manual labour.'

I hate to imagine the workload that would have fallen on Dominique's shoulders. Poor woman.

'However, the village pulled together, and it was agreed that whilst the break healed, Papa would spend his days sitting at the table in the kitchen in our house with his leg up on a bench. Any task from another farm that could be done sitting down would be brought there in the morning for him to work through during the day. In exchange, the others would help Maman with a task on our farm that needed mobility.'

'What a sensible idea.'

'Clothilde and I stayed with Papa to help fetch and carry anything that he needed, and he also set up a little school for us at the other end of the table. He was determined to keep us out of trouble and make sure that we didn't miss out on an education.'

'Was that how Mam's English became so fluent?'

'Absolutely. Papa's French was terrible, even after living here for almost thirty years. He always spoke to me, and therefore your mother, in English. He wasn't a teacher by training, but he loved to tell stories and sing songs, and he played the whistle, so he taught us a lot of old folk tunes.'

Clothilde - 1941

Clothilde is staying the night with Lorna. They are top-to-toe in her bed, and although they can see their breath in the air, they are toasty and warm under the eiderdown.

Rory is wrapped in a blanket and sitting on the floor, with his broken leg stretched out on a sheepskin rug, leaning his back against the door. He is reading to them from a book of Scottish folk tales.

The room is very dark, as the only light is from a candle on the chest of drawers.

'Now girls, are you sure that you want to hear this story? It's one of my favourites, but Dominique thinks that it's too scary for girls your age. It's about the spirit of Almor Burn, which is close to where I grew up.'

Clothilde is not sure whether to speak up. One of the things she likes best about Rory is that he makes her feel safe. The longer she's near him, the more she feels her anxiety subsiding.

Although she doesn't always understand his French, because his vowels are really strange, it's fine when he speaks his own language as he's doing now.

In the end, she answers him in English.

'I don't really like scary stories.'

'Well, this one is a bit scary. How about I just tell you the good bits?'

Both girls cheer in agreement.

Clothilde is glad that Lorna seems as relieved as she is, to have the edited version.

'The tale tonight is of a household spirit that came out of the burn - that's a little stream - and entered the houses in a nearby village, when the people were sleeping.'

Both girls tense up. This is the good version!

'It would go into the houses at night, and walk around, leaving wet footprints all over the floors, as it cleared up any mess the villagers had left behind.'

The girls laugh.

'The people in the village were curious about the visits of this secret night-time helper. They would discuss amongst themselves who might be next to benefit from this helpful spirit. They decided to call it Puddlefoot. But this was a mistake because you mustn't name a household spirit. If you call it directly by name, you will drive it away, and this is what happened.'

The girls are silent, holding their breath to hear what happens next.

'One night a villager came face to face with the spirit and asked if it was Puddlefoot, come to tidy his house. Just like that it vanished, never to be seen again.'

The candle flame gutters for a moment, and one of the girls gasps.

'So, what will you do if you think it has come to visit us here and you're scared?' asks Rory.

'We will shout Puddlefoot!' yelled Lorna.

'Yes, Puddlefoot!' echoes Clothilde as loud as she can.

Isla - 2018

I can conjure up this image in my mind so easily. Rory Stewart sitting in his home entertaining the two young girls with stories of the Scottish Highlands, whilst mending farm machinery or trimming carrots.

It explains so completely how my mother managed to pass for Scottish for the last sixty years.

'Which part of Scotland was your father from Lorna?'

'Da was born in Pitlochry but he only lived there until he was twenty. When war broke out, he joined the Black Watch, and fought with them from the First Battle of the Marne.

Maman was working as a nurse in a regular hospital at the start of the war, but later she worked on the battlefields too, because the male nurses attached to the army couldn't keep up with the number of casualties.

Their paths only crossed for a very brief time, and of course he was with the British army, and she with the French, but Papa was smitten. When the war was over, he came back to find her.'

'That's a beautiful story.'

'It is, although I sometimes wonder if the fairytale nature of it set me up with unrealistic expectations of relationships. I was always looking for a great romance and I never found one, although there were several perfectly nice men I could have married. Is the same true for you, having had Clothilde and James as your parents?'

'Maybe a little. Ma and Da were certainly deeply in love, but I could see how totally absorbing it was for them. There was no space for exploration, either intellectual or geographical. Like Camille, I think I wanted a different life from that of my parents. A life based on the power of my mind. I'm single because I was deeply passionate about my work. Family has never been a major focus in my life. It's very uncharacteristic for me to be here on this search.'

'I'm very glad that you are,' Lorna assures me. 'But why now? What changed?'

'I think it was the shattering of my family construct. I had always thought that I knew it all, and there wasn't much to know. Da was an only child, and my memories of his parents were a bit hazy, as they both died before I was eight. Mam had always told me that she was alone in the world, but she'd given me the impression that she was Scottish born and bred.'

A grin spreads across Lorna's face, in recognition of Mam's nature. At the same time her eyes are full of compassion.

'Discovering that I didn't know who I was, has given me a burning desire to find out the truth.'

'Well, that's wonderful! But so too was following your own path. It took courage and conviction.'

Lorna looks me firmly in the face as she says this.

'It truly is to be admired. Many men, but not many women succeed at doing that.'

I've not known Lorna for very long, but I can tell that she means it.

Sixteen

Isla - 2018

Lorna has invited me back to her apartment, which is above an antique shop. She is eager to show me the handful of photographs that she has from the period before her parents left their farm. She's warned me that there are no photographs of my mother and Camille from the war years, as her parents didn't have access to a camera.

My eye is instantly caught by a familiar image - nestled amongst the books on a shelf beside the front door - Mam, with me as a baby. Pride of place. Lorna's loyal devotion to my mother, is right there, displayed for all to see. How could Mam walk away from her like that?

We enter the living room and Lorna opens an album that she has laid out, ready for us to explore. The first image is of four girls in work clothes. The youngest, my mother, must have been about twelve years old, and the eldest, a blonde girl, looks as if she could possibly have been as much as eighteen.

It's clear that they have been helping with the harvest. Forking hay up onto a cart. The effort of a day's work is shown in the sweat on their faces. But they look as though they are having a great time.

'Who were these two?' I ask, keen to build a picture of my mother's wider circle of friends.

'They moved into the village after the war. Their father arrived looking for work. As neither Papa, nor Joseph, were getting any younger, they scraped together some money to hire him for a few hours each day on both farms. It was a clever move, because with three teenage children - their brother was the one who took the photograph - there were a lot of extra hands on days like this.'

'Mam looks positively radiant.' I point out. 'Why's she so happy?'

'I think her hormones had just kicked in. She was completely head-over-heels for Olivier, the photographer.'

Clothilde - 1948

It's harvest day. The farmers in the area have agreed that the weather should be fair for the next day or two, so Clothilde and her grandparents have been up since first light and are already hard at work in their wheat field.

Clothilde is dressed in her thick, brown, cotton, work skirt, with a smock over the top, and a scarf for her hair. She's glad that she saw sense, and didn't follow the impulse, to wear her sundress with the flowers on.

It's immensely dusty out here in the fields, and scorchingly hot. The stalks of the wheat are totally unforgiving to bare skin and would have scratched her arms to shreds. Luckily the sleeves of the smock are protecting her, as she throws each armful up onto the cart and ties it down.

She much prefers working in the hay fields where the blades of grass are softer and finer. Her grandfather has taught her to use the small scythe, on the condition that she wears the clogs that are currently protecting her feet.

The repetitive twisting motion is fun. It's a bit like dancing when you get it right. However, her favourite bit of harvest is the comfort of the ride home in the hay-cart at the end of the day.

Perhaps this evening she will have the chance to lie side-by-side in a cart with Olivier, as she and her grandparents are due to join his family in the top hayfield for the last few hours of daylight. The hay was cut last night, and it has been left to lie in rows, to dry a little more in today's sun, before being taken to the barn tonight.

Life here in Barantan certainly improved the day that Olivier arrived in the village. He has such wonderful hair. She loves the way it falls across his forehead and covers his left eye, causing him to brush it back in a movement that opens his chest and flexes the muscles of his arm at the same time.

The trouble is that Olivier is not yet showing any sign that he has noticed her, other than as *Lorna's little friend*. It makes her so cross. Especially as for the last few months, she has been just as tall as Lorna.

Isla - 2018

I can see it now. Mam is looking, not at the lens of the camera, but a little above it, in total adoration.

'I think Clothilde's crush lasted until she left the Auvergne, but sadly it was unrequited. Olivier was my age and had plenty of interest from girls in our year at school.'

Another piece of the puzzle falls into place. Olivier must be the young man Mam was talking about at Suncrest that time that she lapsed into dialect.

'Lorna, can I ask you something? When you were growing up, if you weren't using English, did you and Mam speak French or the local dialect?'

'We did both. Maman was keen for us to have opportunities in life, so she insisted we speak French with her, but when we were children amongst ourselves, out in the fields and on the way to school, we weren't going to keep that up - we would have been teased mercilessly.'

I can just imagine how desperate Mam would have been to fit in, with only her grandparents to take her part. Although perhaps Camille was back at this point.

'So did Camille continue working in Vichy after the war, or did she return to Barantan and work the farm?'

Lorna suddenly becomes very still.

'Isla, our conversation this morning took a different turn before I could finish my story about Camille. You were so happy that we'd met. I didn't want to change the mood.'

I can feel an icy lump developing in my chest.

'What happened?'

'As I mentioned, through the winter Camille would come back to see Clothilde on her day off, but it was not unusual for her to miss a week. Personal plans often had to change in wartime. However, in December 1942 Joseph and Chloe became worried. Camille had not been in touch, even by sending word with someone else, for over a month.'

Clothilde - 1942

Clothilde is standing in the gateway at the end of the village, scouring the fields, for a sign of her mother. She is not allowed beyond this point on her own and fear of the Nazis keeps her obedient, but it has been weeks now without contact. Maman must come soon.

She retraces her steps along the lane, but only goes as far as the gate into the vegetable patch. She heads to the drying shed at the far end. She enters, and collects a pair of secateurs, before going back out to the rose bush.

It's an odd spot for a commemorative plant, but the growing conditions are perfect. When they first arrived, Maman had helped her plant a beautiful rose here, for them to remember Papa.

In the early days, Clothilde could recall his face, and his smell, and the sound of his voice, but now that they're no longer in Paris, there are no places that she can go to help her remember. As a result, he is becoming little more than a name in her memory. But he is still a feeling. That comes back whenever she stands here and thinks of him.

The rose has a dead branch that Grand-mère says might have disease. Clothilde was going to ask Maman if they could prune it together on her next visit, but it seems that Maman is not coming. So, it's down to her. She's not going to let Papa's rosebush die!

Slowly she lifts the secateurs to the dead stem. They are heavy and slightly rusted, but eventually they open. She positions the blades around the stem and squeezes. Nothing happens. She places both hands around the handles and squeezes with all her might, but still nothing happens, except for a slight scoring of the bark.

The rage, and desperation at her powerlessness, spill through her defences, and Clothilde throws the offending tool to the ground, knocking over a metal watering-can with a loud clatter, and causing the sheep in the nearby field to flee away, bleating in consternation at the unexpected noise.

The door of the farmhouse opens and at the sight of her grandmother, Clothilde bursts into tears and sinks to the grass.

Chloe rushes out and kneels beside her on the frozen ground, cradling her head in her arms.

'Papa is dead, and now Maman is gone ... I know she is ... and the rosebush is dying too.'

'Oh child, Maman is not dead, they will find her, she will come back.'

Grand-mère says this as if she means it, but lying in her arms on the cold ground, Clothilde can tell that deep down, her grandmother doesn't believe what she's saying. She can feel the lie, in the tension of her grandmother's muscles as she speaks.

With no parents what will happen to her? Will she have to leave? Her grandparents are so busy running the farm. Will they want her if the war ends? Perhaps she can become Lorna's sister? Maybe they will all send her away. But where to?

Clothilde is wracked with sobs, and there is nothing her grandmother can do to console her.

Clothilde is all cried out. She is sitting in front of the fire, wrapped in her grandmother's soft black shawl, a corner of which is grasped tightly in her hand as she sucks her thumb.

She feels exhausted. Her body is quiet and her mind - that has been so busy and hot for many days - now feels empty and clear like a block of ice.

Isla - 2018

I can hardly breathe. The terror at what might have happened to my grandmother is surprisingly real, even though I never knew her.

'She went missing. Was there an accident on the road as she walked here?'

I can't bear the idea of her lying injured in a ditch, alone with little chance of help.

'That was what we thought had happened,' Lorna confirms. 'They asked everyone travelling her route to search the countryside for signs of her. As you can imagine your mother was distraught. She had been living, for the few short hours they had together, whenever Camille was back at the farm.

During those times Clothilde attempted to cling to her like a limpet, but Camille was not a particularly tactile parent, so most of the time Clothilde had to make do with shadowing her mother's every move.'

Mam had never been particularly tactile as a parent herself - that was more Da's style - but I remember how much I had craved her touch. As a child I had taken deliberate steps to engineer situations where contact would be considered natural, and right.

I continued asking her to do things, such as helping me plait my hair before school, long after I was capable of doing it myself.

It wasn't lack of affection. It was just that physical touch wasn't part of her natural repertoire in human interactions. Except with Da of course.

Lorna is speaking once more.

'We finally saw how much Joseph loved his daughter. He spent hours driving the cart, up and down the lanes, and on into Vichy. He was desperately hoping that she had been detained at work.'

'What type of work did Camille actually do?'

'We knew that she had been recruited to work for the Vichy government, based at the town hall, but nobody knew the details. When Joseph asked for her that day, the officials said that there was no-one with her name working there, and that he should go home.'

'They denied her existence?'

'That denial enraged Joseph. So of course, he didn't go home. He needed answers and went looking for them in the only place he could think of. The bakery. He asked if they had seen Camille. Luckily with her sense of style, and the way that she carried herself, she was easy to describe and hard to forget. They remembered her.

For months she had come like clockwork to collect her rations, then suddenly she stopped. They had not seen her in the bakery for more than three weeks.

'Oh my God!' I feel like my insides have suddenly drained out of my feet. 'Did they find her? What happened?'

'No-one knows for sure. The whole village turned out for a more systematic search, but there was no sign of her. The Nazis at this point were making their presence felt in Vichy, and it was dangerous to be seen stirring up trouble, so they couldn't ask too many questions.'

'So, she just vanished? Oh my god. Poor Mam! She was only six.'

I'm too numb to cry. An unexplained disappearance is almost worse than a death. How do you cope with no parents at six years old? An image of Mam as a young child fills my mind, followed by another, of me at the same age with the certain love and fierce protection of my Mam. The thought of having to grow up without Mam, or Da, is unimaginable.

Lorna has started speaking again.

'Quite a long time later, we heard that several members of staff had been taken away for interrogation under suspicion of feeding sensitive information to the allies. It was rumoured that they were shot.'

'And you think Camille was part of this group?'

'Often in such circumstances the Nazis made public spectacles of those who defied them, to function as a deterrent, but no bodies were ever returned to the families, so we were never sure if the story contained any truth.'

'Do you think it likely she would have taken such risks, with Mam to care for?'

'They were exceptional times. Clothilde's nightmares regularly reminded us of Camille's desperation for silence and secrecy as they fled Paris, so I have wondered. But she was a devoted, if slightly brittle mother, especially after Henri's death. She hated being separated from Clothilde. Joseph was furious at the suggestion that his daughter would be so reckless, but I think Chloe's feelings were a more mixed. I detected a hint of pride at the suggestion that her daughter might be that brave. Although Chloe never got over her disappearance.'

I nod. Right now, I know how she feels.

The shock of this news has deeply affected me, and I didn't even know Camille. All I can think about is my poor mother. Uprooted from her home, and any connections she had formed in Paris. Brought to a tiny village, and a rural life she didn't understand. To be told that her beloved father was dead, and then suffer almost immediate separation from her mother, when she was forced to work in Vichy. It's no surprise at all that anxiety became Mam's most significant character trait.

Living in such a heightened, and prolonged state of anxiety must've had a devastating impact on the development of such a young child. Especially during wartime.

For this to be followed, only two years later, by the permanent disappearance of her remaining parent, must surely have created a mental fracturing from which she could never recover.

How dangerous to love. How dangerous to trust. How dangerous to hope.

'Lorna, would you mind if we looked at the rest of the photographs tomorrow?'

I close the albums and place them in a pile as I push my chair back.

'I'm feeling quite upset, and I'd like to go back to my hotel room and process everything that you've told me.'

'Of course,' Lorna places her hand over mine. 'This is the first time you've heard all of this. I still feel it, and I have known it all my life. I am very sorry to have been the bearer of such sad news.'

Clothilde - 1942

Clothilde is sitting on her bed with her back against the wall. Hugging her knees, as she stares across at the twin bed opposite. Maman's bed. Its presence - in the room that they are supposed to share - has dominated her thoughts, and dreams, every night since her grandparents gave her the news that her mother was missing.

She is desperate to drag it from the room. Just to have the chance to pretend that Maman is downstairs, or out feeding the chickens, and will be back at any moment. A bed that hasn't been slept in, screams out *I should be here, but I'm gone. I've left you. I'm not coming back.*

Of course, Maman has not been sleeping here regularly for the last couple of years, but her smell would always last on the pillow between visits. When Clothilde was missing her, she could climb into the bed herself, and bury her face in the pillow. Breathing in her mother's scent, she had always felt comforted and reassured.

Now the scent is gone. Even though she has refused to let Grand-mère wash the bedding.

Clothilde can feel the cold clear ice spreading from her brain, down through her body, around her heart, and into the pit of her stomach. Her ears feel slightly muffled, as if she is under water, and she is certain, that fairly soon, she too will be gone. Frozen into a statue. Locking out the pain.

Seventeen

Isla - 2018

When I woke up this morning, I didn't feel able to take any more bad news. I was considering phoning Lorna to cancel my visit. However, I realised that I needed to hear how Mam pulled through. Because somehow, she did cope without her mother.

So now, I am back here at Lorna's apartment.

As she shows me into her front room, I catch sight of a beautifully decorated Easter egg on the windowsill - a fine example of the style Mam and I used to try every year when I was growing up.

'I didn't notice this yesterday. It's gorgeous. Did you make it yourself?'

'Yes, I make one every year. It's more difficult to blow the eggs and do the fine paintwork these days, as my arthritis is pretty bad, but I make the effort in honour of my family. It was something that we used to do together every Easter.'

'Did you teach Mam?'

I think back to the occasions around our own kitchen table in Scotland, when Mam would sit me down with a pin, and an egg, with instructions to blow gently through the tiny hole so that all the contents, would slide out of the egg into the waiting bowl, through the larger hole that I had made in the bottom.

'Mam taught me when I was little too. It was always my favourite craft activity because it came with built-in scrambled eggs for breakfast. Mind you, ours were never as beautiful as your one.'

'We did teach your mother to blow eggs, but not until after the war, as we didn't have access to the paints for decorating. However, we did still celebrate Easter with coloured eggs. We would hard-boil them with beetroot, or red onion peelings in the water, so that the shells turned purple. It was a real treat to have a whole egg each.'

As Lorna speaks, I realise that some of the stories that I'd heard yesterday, had come from a time after Camille's disappearance, and yet I hadn't guessed. They were just stories of a regular little girl growing up in wartime. It's obvious that I have Lorna's family to thank for the laughter, and day-to-day pleasures, in Mam's life.

Lorna gestures for me to sit at the table with her, so that we can look at the remaining photographs.

'From everything you've told me, it sounds as if Mam was never very close to Joseph and Chloe. I guess it's hard to take on a small child when you're older. I know it's not something that I would welcome at this stage in my life, and of course they were grieving the death of their own daughter.'

'Oh, no, you've got it wrong. They loved Clothilde very much. After the war they spent a lot of time with her, helping her discover school subjects that made the most of her talents, and activities that were fun for her to do at home, despite the lack of people her own age in the area.'

My heart lifts. Mam had people who loved her.

'The war years were terrible for everyone, and the truth is that things weren't much better in the years that followed. Life on the farm was unrelenting back-breaking work, but the village understood that and pulled together to support Chloe and Joseph in their new role as surrogate parents.'

Lorna is very animated in defence of her old neighbours.

'The stories you are hearing are of course just *my* memories of Clothilde. Chloe and Joseph would have had their own. You have to remember that my parents were already keeping an eye out for me, so it was easier for all the adults, if Clothilde and I were together. It was also more fun for us.'

I smile to assure her that I've understood.

'So, what did Mam like doing?'

I'm curious to develop my picture of the young Clothilde.

'She was a daredevil on a bicycle!'

This comes as a surprise, as Mam was incredibly risk averse during my childhood.

'I think it started during the war. We had one bike in the village, and she and I would often borrow it, to take messages for people. Sometimes we were also asked to deliver things. As I was bigger, I usually did the pedalling standing up. Your Mam would handle the package. Balancing herself whilst sitting on the seat, standing on the back carrier bracket, or sitting on the handlebars, depending on the odd shaped item we were delivering.'

I love this image. It's so full of the exuberance of youth and has so little to do with the rather constrained mother I grew up with.

'She also loved all forms of needlework - embroidery, knitting, crocheting, and even dressmaking.'

Now this is the mother I know. Until she moved into Suncrest Mam always had a needlework project of some sort on the go.

'Chloe helped her to make several outfits for special occasions. Clothilde even made me a dress one summer, because I wanted Emil to notice me.'

'Emil? Who was he?'

'Oh, just a boy at school. His family left the area when I was sixteen. That happened a lot after the war. One week he was there and the next he was gone.'

A look of deep sadness crosses Lorna's face, and I wonder if Emil, for her, was the one that got away.

Clothilde - 1946

Clothilde and Lorna have come to the market in Le Vernet to find some material for a dress. It's got to be special. There are two stalls that sell cloth. This one has a beautiful piece of sky-blue silk, but there is no way that Lorna can afford it. Apart from this, they've got nothing unusual. So, all hopes must now be pinned on the stall at the far end.

As they walk down between the rows, Clothilde can't help being drawn to the fruit stalls. She's never seen fruit in such abundance. Dominique warned her what to expect this morning, but it was impossible to imagine.

Apparently, this is what every market was like before the war. Peaches and apricots, plums and cherries, raspberries and strawberries, all available to buy. It makes her feel dizzy. The years of rationing are truly over.

As they approach the end of the row, she can see large bolts of cloth draped over a high-sided cart. The top layers are all heavy weight cotton, suitable for work clothes but, peeping through from underneath, Clothilde spots a flash of primrose yellow.

She hurries forward and begins to wrestle with the oversized bolts. The stall owner is quick to help her, and soon yards and yards, of beautiful, delicate, summer weight cotton, are pouring across the cart like a burst of sunshine.

'This is it!' Clothilde says as she wraps one end around her friend's shoulders. 'It's perfect with your dark hair, and there is no way Emil can miss you when you walk into the dance.'

Isla - 2018

We turn our attention to the pile of photographs.

'Who are these two?' I ask, of a pair of older men, sitting in front of a bar drinking beer.

'That is my father and Joseph, your great-grandfather.'

I smile. It's a great image. So French, and yet one of them still manages to have the look of his Scottish origins.

'It was taken the year before he died.'

'Who died?'

'Joseph.'

'No!' My breath catches in my throat. More death for Mam.

'He developed severe breathing problems in late 1947. He'd been a heavy smoker all his life, and probably had lung cancer. Anyway, his condition deteriorated quickly, and he died in spring of 1948. He was only fifty-eight.'

'So, what happened to Chloe and Mam? Could they manage the farm alone?'

I don't see how they could have.

'Olivier, who by this time was fifteen, had decided to leave school to work on the farm full time. So, he took over the day-to-day tasks under Chloe's instruction, but they all knew it wasn't a long term solution. Even though we were farming our two properties as if they were one, the two together still weren't viable.'

'Would you and Mam have wanted to take over if they had been?'

'Aside from the fact that we were girls, and that wasn't ever thought to be an option, no, I wanted to go into teaching, and at the time your mother was more interested in a career in nursing. We muddled along for a few more years, but it all came to a head once Chloe knew she was dying.'

I am horrified.

'You mean that Mam lost both her parents, and both the grandparents that she lived with, by the time she was fifteen?'

Lorna nods.

It's a staggering level of loss. I can't believe that I'd been oblivious to it all. Of course, I knew that Mam's parents had died before I was born, but somehow, I had always assumed that she'd had them for longer.

Even in recent days, I had created a whole fantasy in which Mam's grandparents saw her through to adulthood, and maybe even had a chance to meet Da. Now I realise that this was incredibly far from the truth.

My gaze returns to the image of Rory and Joseph so happy together.

'Have you got a photograph of Chloe?' I ask hopefully.

'I wish I had a good one. She appears in the background in a lot of the pictures that I've got. She was always very shy of the camera, as she believed she was ugly, but I always thought she had a rather handsome face. She had these lovely, friendly, crinkles around her eyes.'

Lorna passes me a group photograph, possibly taken the same summer as the picture in the hayfield. There are about fifteen people, of assorted ages, arranged in a gateway. Some of the younger ones are sitting on the top bar of the gate, the older adults standing in front, and a couple of young lads are lying on the ground at their feet.

'That's Chloe.' Lorna points to the woman in the centre.

She appears to have streaked grey hair, swept back, and tied into a bun at the nape of her neck. I peer closely, but the image isn't large enough to see the crinkles that Lorna mentioned. However, she is looking fondly across at Mam, who is making a sweeping gesture with her arm, her mouth wide open, obviously caught in raucous laughter by the photographer, before she was ready.

'It looks like she and Mam had a nice relationship.'

'They did. They eventually became very close. Especially after Joseph died.'

'What happened to Chloe? She doesn't look that old here.'

'You're right. She was only fifty-five when she died. The malnutrition and heavy labour around the farm during the war had taken a lot out of her, so when there was a bad outbreak of influenza in the village, she couldn't shake it off.'

'The flu? That seems such an insignificant condition to die from, we catch it all the time and recover.'

'People in farming communities are notorious for avoiding the doctor, and as I mentioned, they think that her system was weakened by long-term malnutrition. You may not realise it, but people still die every year from the flu even now.'

'Do they?' I'm astonished. 'In Europe?'

Lorna nods.

'I had no idea.'

Clothilde - 1951

Clothilde is sitting beside her grandmother's bed holding her hand. This can't be happening. She's so ill. There *has* to be a way to make her better. The damp flannel lying across her forehead, is only staying cool for a matter of moments before her raging temperature heats it through.

She hasn't eaten anything for three days and is only taking tiny sips of water.

At times she's able to talk, but most of the time, when the fever grips, she makes no sense at all. Perhaps she is hallucinating?

The door opens and Dominique enters.

'Clothilde, let me sit with her for a moment. Go down to the kitchen and have something to eat with Rory. I've made a stew. You need to keep your strength up, otherwise you will catch it too.'

Clothilde reluctantly heads to the kitchen.

Rory is sitting at the table with two bowls ready filled. He pats the table and gestures for her to come and join him.

'Clothilde, I need to talk to you. A few days ago, when Chloe first became ill, but before things got this bad, she asked for my help. She asked that I help her write to your father's family in Brittany, to ask them to take you in if anything happens to her.'

'No!'

Clothilde's shriek is piercing. A direct representation of the overwhelming pain of every earlier separation and loss.

'Don't send it. She won't die.' The tears are pouring down her face. 'I can stay with you, in Lorna's room. She won't mind.'

'Clothilde, this is the hardest conversation I have ever had to have. You know how much we love you, but Lorna is going to study teaching next year, and with your grandfather gone, and neither farm doing well, Dominique and I have to sell.'

'Sell?'

'There are men who want to buy our land, to build houses. They are offering a lot of money, and we are too old to continue to farm on our own.'

'So, you won't be living here? But what will happen if Grand-mère recovers?'

'We have been discussing the land offer together in recent weeks. We all plan to move to Le Vernet. There are some small houses there, and with the money from selling the farms we can retire there and be close to each other.'

Clothilde is clutching at straws.

'Then we can still do that, even if she dies.'

'Clothilde you are not old enough to live alone, and I'm very sorry, but you can't move in with us. The houses are too small, and Dominique is facing new responsibility for her parents who are unwell. She will be spending much of her time with them, and I am not able to take care of you alone.'

'Why not?' Clothilde pushes her chair back violently. 'You looked after me most of my childhood.'

'That was different.'

Clothilde is too angry and hurt to acknowledge the way that Rory's fists are clenched so tightly, that his nails will leave groove marks in his palms, or the deep pain that crosses his face, as he continues to speak.

'This is your grandmother's decision. She has thought about it very deeply, and she handles your care.'

Isla - 2018

I can't take my eyes off my great-grandmother's image. What a tragedy to die so young. Only a little older than I am now. That's quite a thought!

'So did Mam move in with you when Chloe died?'

It seems the obvious arrangement.

'No, unfortunately that didn't happen. When Chloe realised that my parents were not going to be able to take Clothilde to Le Vernet with them, she asked Papa to search Camille's belongings for the address in Brittany of Henri's family. Chloe had been storing her daughter's possessions, for Clothilde, in the original suitcases Camille had brought with her from Paris.'

I think of the strong leather case in my parents' attic. Perhaps it had belonged to Camille. I wish I'd known. I would have kept it.

'Chloe and Joseph had always been set against that whole family. Especially as none of them had written during the war years. However, despite this, Chloe intended to beg them to take Clothilde.'

'Oh, no! Not another forced separation! I'd always assumed that you and Mam just grew apart when you started your adult lives.'

'I wish it had been that way. Then maybe she would have stayed in touch. Unfortunately, what happened caused a breach that never fully healed.'

I can see the deep anguish of years of separation, behind Lorna's eyes.

'There was very little time to make the arrangements. Chloe found the strength to write the letter but didn't want to speak to Clothilde until she had definite news about her future. She knew that uncertainty and separations were both extremely hard for her granddaughter, and she hoped to make the steps of the transition as clear as possible for her. Regrettably she slipped into semi-delirium long before the reply came from Brittany.'

Tears are welling in Lorna's eyes as she speaks.

'Two weeks after the funeral, we drove Clothilde to Vichy, and watched her board a train to Brittany. It was the last time we ever saw her.'

Clothilde - 1951

Clothilde steps down onto the Parisian platform carrying her satchel and large leather suitcase. Crowds of passengers are alighting from trains all around her. It's overwhelming.

Her breathing has become shallow and is getting faster. Memories of her last time at this station come flooding in. Grasping the hem of her mother's coat. Terrified that they would lose each other in the mayhem. Desperately trying to avoid stumbling over this very same leather case, as its heavy weight caused it to swing erratically from her mother's hand.

Now, more than ten years later she is back. Alone. What good have those years done her. Every person that she invested in is either dead or has rejected her. Life is no different than if she had just let go of her mother's coattails that day and been swallowed up by the crowd.

Rory Stewart had continued his meddling letter writing - asking the railway company to help her make this journey. He'd reminded them that Henri had been killed at work and suggested that they had an obligation to assist.

An official reply had refused, but someone, perhaps a friend of her father's, had taken unofficial action, because a few days later an envelope had arrived containing a ticket to Paris, the details of a boarding house in the city, and another ticket for her onward journey to St Pierre Quiberon tomorrow.

Perhaps it's returning to her father's place of work, but, for the first time in twelve years she has a clear sense of who he was.

It's as much a feeling as an image. Her father carrying her up the stairs to their apartment. It was always very late at night after they had all spent an evening out visiting friends. Her parents would often put her to bed wherever they were and wake her up when it was time to go home.

She would wake to the familiar smell of cigarettes that clung to his hair, and the feeling of her father's arms around her, as he scooped her up out of the unfamiliar bed to make the journey home.

A lump forms in her throat, and she can feel unfamiliar tears brimming in her eyes. She has not cried once since Grand-mère died. The ice has returned, and until this moment, she had been certain it would never thaw.

She wonders what brand of cigarettes Papa used to smoke, because that smell had always made her feel safe. She wishes she could smell it now because this city is terrifying.

Oh, for that innocent certainty she'd had the last time she was here, that her father was still alive.

As Rory had suggested, she takes her luggage straight across town to Gare Montparnasse, so that she can leave it overnight in their left luggage office. It is then much easier to continue on foot to her boarding house.

It doesn't look promising. The paint is peeling on the weather-beaten street door, but the plaque on the wall confirms that she's in the right place. She pushes the door and enters a small courtyard. On the far side is another door leading to a set of stairs. As she appears into the light of the courtyard, a woman leans from an upstairs window to enquire what business she has there.

It's not long before Clothilde is in a tiny room that faces the street. The daylight is fading, and although Rory made sure that she had enough money to get herself a meal in a restaurant, she is too scared to go out alone in the dark.

She still has some bread and cheese left over from lunchtime. She'd wrapped it that morning in one of her grandfather's handkerchiefs, so that he would be with her on her journey. She's glad to have those memories now, in this unsettling room, as she perches on the edge of the bed to eat.

Clothilde's courage is all but gone. It has been a shock to realise that she has only herself to rely on. She's not sure what type of establishment this is, but there have been people coming and going all evening, with lots of knocking on doors and speaking in hushed tones in the hall.

She can hear someone coming down the corridor towards her room.

It's too much. She jumps out of the bed and gives it a shove, so that it slides across in front of the door. It makes a terrible shrieking noise on the floorboards, but she doesn't care.

She needs to prevent people from entering without her knowledge as she sleeps. She climbs back into the bed, puts her head under the pillow, and hopes for the best.

Isla - 2018

The depth of Mam's tragedy just keeps opening like a trap door below me. I feel numb, as though I have no emotions left.

'We wanted to have her back for visits, but I don't think she could forgive us for following Chloe's wishes and sending her away.'

'Surely it was no surprise that she wanted to stay with you all?'

The moment I've spoken I wish I could take it back. That sounded so harsh. Lorna's head recoils defensively, but she ignores my comment, and struggles on with her explanation.

'Of course we knew, but I had finished school and was going away to study, and the farms were sold for development. Life was changing for all of us.'

I swallow hard.

'Did she know these people?'

'No, and I'm afraid I don't even know their names, let alone the part of Brittany in which they lived. Clothilde and I did write for a while, but I always copied the return address directly from her envelope.'

This is not looking good.

'Do you think that the name of my grandfather's family, Marec, is a common one?'

'I wouldn't know, but Brittany is vast. You will need something else to narrow down your search.'

And there it is, another dead end.

My month of annual leave is nearly up and tomorrow I must say goodbye to Lorna. I've got so used to seeing her every day, sharing a meal, or a glass of wine, sitting quietly enjoying each other's company. It will be a huge wrench to leave.

My only consolation is the discovery that Lorna uses email and is keen to explore video chat. I probably have her career in teaching to thank for the fact that, at eighty-five, she is still keeping up with technological developments.

It's odd that Lorna is the one who has finally helped me to understand, what it feels like to have family. Perhaps it's because she willingly shared such deeply personal and emotional family history. In contrast to my parents, who found it so difficult to talk to me about their past.

Maybe the closeness that has developed between us, is because in some way, for her, I've taken my mother's place. I know that I have a little of that feeling in reverse, and I like it. However, we have talked about death so much in recent weeks that I'm acutely aware of her age.

Although she seems in relatively good health right now, at eighty-five, it cannot last forever. I mustn't leave it too long before visiting again. I can't afford to repeat the mistake that I made with Mam.

I park my rental car outside Lorna's building, and having rung the bell, I return to lean on the car in the sunshine, as she makes her way slowly down. We agreed last night that we wouldn't prolong this moment. Just a brief farewell to send me on my way.

However, as I stand here now, I'm realising what a terrible idea that was. Why didn't we have a long breakfast together whilst we had the chance? The door opens and her hunched frame appears, with the now familiar bent kneed twist to meet my gaze.

Her eyes crinkle, and a smile spreads across her face, as she strides purposefully towards me with the aid of her stick. My heart melts at the sight. Some people would be defeated by this level of curvature and painful arthritis, but not Lorna. Her lively and indefatigable personality mean that, certainly in public, she shows little sign of obstacle.

I want to hug her, but I haven't thought this through. It would be easier if we were both sitting down. In the end I settle for a kiss on the cheek but open the car door, so that later I can sit for a final farewell hug.

'Lorna, I don't know how to begin to thank you for these last few weeks.' I struggle to get the words out. 'It's been a delight to get to know you, and you've given me an understanding of my mother that will radically transform every memory that I have of her. You've provided me with a gateway to compassion, and hopefully a better understanding of myself.'

'Oh, my child, that's nothing to what you've given me. Not only did you add the joy of your beautiful self to my life. You brought your mother back as well, through all those stories of your life in Scotland, and through every movement that you made. She is echoed in the way you hold your limbs, and the fleeting expressions on your face.'

She reaches out and caresses my cheek as she speaks.

'Above all else, you confirmed for me that her decision to cut herself off was the right one for her. That you lived your life, unaware of her past, is proof that she found a way to exist, without the constant anguish that had formed the background of her early life. For that, my own sadness has been a small price to pay.'

Tears form beneath my eyelashes as I hear the desolation and personal tragedy in what Lorna is saying. Her capacity for benevolence, and generosity of spirit, towards her childhood friend is remarkable.

'We will stay in touch, won't we?' I ask plaintively as I lower myself into the car.

Lorna reaches in and gives me the hug that I have so longed for.
'Without a doubt my dear. Drive safely.'

Was Lorna right? Did Mam find a way, with Da's help, to silence her inner terrors and live in peace? Mam's life certainly wasn't anxiety free. Far from it. I know that there were times when she had terrible nightmares, because I would hear voices late at night, and Da going downstairs a short while later to make hot milk for her.

I asked him about it once, but he just reminded me that I had nightmares too from time to time, and that it was nothing to worry about, and so I didn't.

I need to stop in Vichy for petrol and realise that I can't leave the area without at least trying to understand the city, and what happened here during the war.

I take out my phone to search for the local war museum, but there isn't one. I'm surprised. In Germany, whenever I've been to areas with political, wartime significance they have always contained museums.

It seems that the citizens of Vichy are not yet accepting of their past. Without the help of a museum, I turn to the Internet in search of explanations. It's difficult to reconcile the spa town that I can see today, with its complicated history.

What I discover causes my feminist hackles to rise. At the time when Camille and Mam were fleeing the Nazi invasion of Paris, Pétain was heading up the Vichy government in free- France. They were intent on implementing a National Revolution of their own.

Swapping 'liberté, égalité, fraternité' ('freedom, equality, fraternity') for 'famille, travaille, patrie' ('family, work, nation').

A woman's place, as far as they were concerned, was back in the home. However, this didn't last long, as the lack of men in the labour force resulted in many women like Camille taking up positions within the administration.

There followed an era of total hypocrisy amongst government officials - preaching family values, and penalising those who did not adhere to their official moral code, whilst living debauched lifestyles themselves.

It is this environment that Camille endured daily at work. I can imagine - glamorous as she was - that she would have caught the eye of many high-ranking officials.

This would have been an advantage if there were any truth to the rumour that she was working for the resistance, but either way, a minefield to navigate as a woman in a male-dominated high-stakes environment. It's no surprise that this culture of lies and double standards resulted in the cover-up of the circumstances surrounding her departure from the town hall.

The Vichy government also wanted the population back on the land, away from urban prosperity and intellectual advancement. So, they came up with the slogan 'retournez à la terre '('return to the soil').

According to these articles women and girls were not supposed to work the land either. Their choices were meant to be limited to the 'feminine skills'.

However, once again, needs must in wartime. Mam and Lorna laboured away, just like the boys in the area, and as far as I can see, they both carried out their tasks extremely well.

The real change came on 10th November 1942 when the Nazis arrived in Vichy. It was very soon after this that Camille disappeared, and from that time until the end of the war, every resident of Barantan lived under the threat of Nazi punishment.

Eighteen

Isla - 2018

My apartment feels cold and empty. For so many years, all that I needed to feel ok was this tranquil bubble away from work. An elegant, uncluttered space, where all my senses could relax.

Now, it seems that I'm missing human company. The homely jumble in Lorna's apartment, had strongly echoed the environment of my childhood home, and recreated the feeling of life with my parents.

Our kitchen table strewn with papers, or the preparations for cooking. Bags of knitting on the sofa - ready for Mam's idle hands. Fishing rods and hiking poles spilling out of the umbrella stand by the front door. Although my return to the office tomorrow will reconnect me with people, it's my specific humans whose company I yearn for.

My month away has definitely done me good. I'm back to my usual work rate, and my mind is more focused, now that so many questions regarding my mother's life have been answered.

However, during these last few weeks back in Dortmund other things are noticeably changing. Throughout my career I've relished the challenges of the corporate world. I've been proud to achieve company goals, and often exceeded the expectations of my colleagues.

I've enjoyed the travel, financial security, and sense of accomplishment. But being a resolute leader, an efficient manager and a loyal company employee is no longer enough.

I have a yearning for more breadth and meaning to my existence. I've begun wearing the more casual clothes that I bought in Scotland and taking regular walks to think about my life and what I want for myself.

It's not realistic to think that I will suddenly have time to join clubs, or classes, in the evenings, or even at weekends, as my workload hasn't diminished. But scheduling regular holidays would be a good commitment to life outside the office.

I've also resolved to leave work at the office. So, whilst I stay late most evenings, once I eventually return to my apartment, the time is my own.

It is time for my second Professional Development Meeting. Peter is looking at me expectantly with a slight sparkle in his eye.

'So, before we start the official stuff. How are you? The time off seems to have done you good.'

'It did. I spent the whole time in the Auvergne, where I met Mam's best friend, Lorna. She's in her eighties. She's the most incredible woman.'

'I can see what an impression the trip has made on you, Isla. You're glowing with happiness.'

I hear what he is saying and immediately feel guilty.

'Peter, I've given you the wrong impression. It was horrendous. Every day I learnt of further heartbreak. Mam had a desperately sad childhood. I don't know why I'm behaving as if I've returned from a package holiday to Greece.'

'Isla I don't think your happiness is based on what you learnt in France, I think it's the result of having found a friend.'

I stop talking and stare at him. It's deeply frustrating that this man has more insight into my personality than I have myself. Although it's too soon to call Peter a friend, we have always had a very open, straight-talking relationship in the office.

The truth is that with my lack of human connections elsewhere, he knows me better than anyone else on the planet.

Seeing that he has flummoxed me with his almost telepathic thoughts, Peter changes the subject and begins our meeting.

'Isla, now that you're back I have something that I would like you to consider. We discussed the need for you to have a new challenge.'

'Yes,' I say hesitantly, unsure what will follow.

'Whilst you were away I was given a promotion.'

'Congratulations!' I interrupt enthusiastically.

Peter manages to look simultaneously delighted and dismissive, by nodding and making smoothing motions with his hands.

'Officially I will be based here, but I am going to have a lot of other responsibilities off site, so I will be looking for someone to take the role of my deputy. It won't relate to any of the technical side, just the line-management and I can't think of anyone more suitable than you.'

I sit still, expecting the flush of success that has accompanied past promotions. To my surprise, and Peter's, it doesn't arrive.

'What's the matter?' he asks.

'I'm not sure. Normally I get a fizz of adrenaline and an instant flood of ideas. Don't get me wrong. I like the thought of stepping up and collaborating more closely with you. I'm just surprised by my response. When will the job be advertised?'

'I can probably give you a couple of weeks to think about it.'

Back at home I change into walking gear and head for the river to think. A year ago, I would have been over the moon if I'd been offered the additional role of senior onsite executive in Dortmund. So why not today? I know that I can do it, but there is no driving energy, no acceleration towards the new target, no excitement for the future.

Instead, I'm wondering how Lorna is getting on back in Le Vernet, and what I should cook this evening when I get home.

The golf club is holding a memorial event for Da on the anniversary of his death, this weekend, and they would like me to be there. Whilst it's short notice, there is no practical reason why I shouldn't go.

However, I'm not sure how I feel at the prospect of being back in West Kilbride without my parents. It seems unbelievably pathetic. Mam had to deal with this situation from the age of six. Surely at fifty-three I can manage it.

Maybe I sold the house too quickly? Perhaps I should have waited until I'd had more of a chance to grieve, to sit in their home, to be with their things? The hard truth, is that the new me, is the one that wants this. The Isla of six months ago just saw the financial drain and awkward practicalities of handling an empty house, miles from where she lived.

I've been determined not to give up my hunt for Mam's family. In my spare time I have been searching the genealogy databases for references to the name Marec, based in Brittany, but it has proved impossible. There are so many of them, that without a birth certificate for Henri I'm stuck.

I think I *will* go back to Scotland this weekend. It will be a nice distraction from the frustrations of my search. I can go to the memorial with Andrew, and then make my way up to Loch Lomond for an overnight stay, before returning to work.

I've not been back to the loch since I was a teenager, and I would like to revisit the area now that I've read my father's letters. I think seeing it through his eyes will help me feel close to both my parents.

It's a day of squally showers. Quite fitting really for Da. The weather never stopped him from heading out. I heed his oft-repeated advice, and dress appropriately for the weather rather than the occasion.

Over my smart black trousers and cream silk blouse I add a black cashmere cardigan, a pair of navy waterproof trousers and a bright red rain jacket. I leave behind the black court shoes, and instead put on the black leather ankle boots that I brought for hiking tomorrow. Nice and dry despite the occasional sudden downpour on my walk to join Andrew.

He takes one look at me and bursts out laughing.

'You're back!' he almost shouts in delight, throwing his arms wide.

'What do you mean?' I ask, confused. He only saw me half an hour ago as I'm staying at his house.

'This is the Isla I remember! When you were a little girl, you were always playing by a rockpool in your raincoat and wellies. Whatever the weather. James' little shadow.'

I smile in recognition. He's right. I always wanted to be where Da was. I never expected him to play with me, although he often did. I just liked to be in his orbit when he wasn't working.

'Well, I've not changed that much. My smart outfit's underneath!'

'Leave your raingear on for now, we're about to go out to the spot where he passed away. We'll say a few words out there on the course and then come back here and drink a toast.'

I get a sudden sinking feeling at the thought of going out onto the fairway. I clutch onto a nearby chair for support. It's not as if it will be my first time there, or that I didn't know the plan. My reaction has taken me by surprise.

'Come on kid, hang on to me.' Andrew says crossing the room and offering me his arm. 'I could do with the support myself.'

And so, we head out into the rain arm-in-arm.

It's been an emotional day, and fond as I am of Andrew, I need a little time to myself. Once again, I'm standing alone on our rock. The light this evening - after all the rain earlier in the day - is beautiful. It's a phenomenon that I've noticed many times. It has an inexplicable, washed-clean quality.

At this time of year, it barely gets dark before the dawn breaks again. Da and I always loved to watch the way that the light and the water interact with changing intensity as the sun goes down. We would stand here on many evenings, long past my bedtime, enjoying the beauty of nature.

I wish I could talk to him now. I need his quiet, supportive form of guidance. In all our years together, he never once told me what to do, but he was always on hand to help me unravel the tangled netting of any problem. I would use his still presence as a sounding board, and he would ask the occasional pertinent question to gently remind me who I am.

Who I am. Is that the same as who I was? That little girl in rain gear on the beach. How did she become the high-flying business executive? Curiosity and drive, and the need for a challenge. But what happened to slow observation, to the connections to nature, and the search for beauty?

I must give Peter an answer about the job in a couple of days, but it seems impossible to step forward in any direction. Peter was right when he identified that I have outgrown my current role. There is nothing left in it for me.

The deputy position would be new, with a wider international scope across the company. However, I would have little autonomy as Peter's number two. It would be an option to look elsewhere for a challenge, but I have no enthusiasm for a new role in a new company.

In fact, the only thing that energises me at the moment is my desire to understand my family.

Mam provided me with multiple, incoherent clues during her last months at Suncrest, and Lorna has shared her own set of incomplete memories from their childhood together. Unfortunately, I feel as though I've shoved them all in the same bag, to get tangled up together. Oh, for Da's ability to unravel a problem.

This morning, Andrew and I are eating toast in his kitchen, when he suddenly jumps up and runs out of the room shouting.

'The package. I'm an idiot!'

A moment later he returns with a small packet wrapped in newspaper and tied together with string.

'I found this last week after we spoke. I knew I'd be seeing you, so I didn't bother to call again. I can't believe I nearly forgot!' He hands me the parcel.

'Where was it?' I'm confused.

'That wonderful desk that belonged to your parents.'

'What?'

'Come on I'll show you.'

He jumps up again. Curious I follow him into the front room, where the desk now has pride of place under the window. He pulls out the supports and folds down the flap that becomes the writing surface, revealing the little pigeonholes for envelopes and other forms of stationary and writing paraphernalia.

'Didn't we open the lid?'

I say thinking back to the day when Andrew collected it, and we took all the big drawers out to get it in the car.

'I'm surprised you haven't used it until now.'

'Oh, no.' Andrew shakes his head 'I've used the desk a lot. The packet wasn't in one of the pigeonholes, it was in here.' And with that he reaches forward and presses on the back panel of one of the shallower pigeonholes. The whole panel comes away in his hand revealing a large cavity.

'Spring-loaded!' he says with delight.

'Wow! A secret compartment.'

I'm stunned by the amazing craftsmanship.

'How on earth did you discover it?'

'A once in a lifetime attempt at dusting. I was thinking of your parents, and feeling guilty that I wasn't looking after their beautiful desk. This discovery was the result of a crisis of conscience.'

'If only I'd known about this as a child. It would have been such fun!'

I have a twinge of regret at the lost opportunity, before pulling myself together.

'Shall we go back and see what's in the packet?'

We return to the kitchen and with care, as the paper is old, I open the packet, revealing multiple, handwritten letters. Many with French stamps. All addressed to Mam.

The tears of joy and relief pour down my face.

Andrew, thinking that I'm upset, stands, and comes around to my side of the table so that he can put his arm around me.

I hurry to explain.

'I thought I was at a dead end.' I sniff, grinning from ear to ear. 'With these letters there's hope again'.

'Isla, I'm lost. What are you talking about?'

'There's so much that's gone on in the last few months that I haven't yet told you Andrew. As you know I've been trying to trace Mam's past in France.'

Andrew lets go of my shoulder and sits back down ready for an update.

'Mam left the Auvergne when she was fourteen and I had no way to follow her journey after that, as Lorna no longer had the address.'

I pick up the bundle of letters and reach out with them towards Andrew.

'But look at these stamps, these are letters written to Mam from France! The envelopes have return addresses on them, and see, this one says Bretagne - Brittany. I'll be able to continue my search!'

Andrew smiles but it fades quickly.

'So will these letters all be written in French?'

'Oh, I hadn't thought about that, yes I suppose they will.'

My shoulders slump. I've let my French lapse as Lorna and I were so happy speaking English together, and I never did get as far as multiple tenses and extended vocabulary.

Andrew notices my deflation and hurries to share his solution.

'Why don't you pop down to Suncrest and see if Elspeth has a forwarding address for Adjavella? Everybody loved her, so they're bound to have kept in touch.'

I'm overwhelmed by remorse. Why don't I have Adjavella's contact details myself? She did so much for Mam, and for me at the worst time in my life, and yet I just walked away without a thought.

Who was I back then?

I readily cut people from my life in an instant with the precise incision worthy of a surgeon.

'You could send Adjavella the letters,' Andrew continues. 'I'm sure she would translate them for you. She was really fond of Tilly, and she's bound to be just as keen to find out about Tilly's past as you are.'

I can feel a warmth flooding through me at this solution. There is no one I would rather share this search with than Adjavella.

I glance at my phone. There's just time to run down the hill to the care home before my train to Glasgow. Hopefully Elspeth will be on duty. It would be nice to see her. I don't know why I didn't think of dropping by yesterday. In fact, I've done it again. I should have suggested that Andrew invite Elspeth to Da's memorial. After all, she spent many hours with him at Suncrest whilst he was visiting Mam.

I'm so ashamed. My thought processes just don't seem to automatically include other people, or their connections to each other.

I push open the door and step into the, all too familiar, reception area. There behind the desk is Elspeth. She looks up and greets me with a huge beaming smile. I'm not used to eliciting that response in other people, and for a minute it's overwhelming.

She hurries around the desk and opens her arms to hug me.

'Isla, you're back!'

'Only briefly, but it's wonderful to see you Elspeth!' I hug her back. 'Sadly, this is a flying visit, as I'm leaving for Loch Lomond in an hour, but I had to come and say hello, and I must admit I'm also hoping to ask a favour.'

'Of course,' Elspeth says returning to her seat behind the desk and gesturing to me to pull up another. 'What can I do?'

'This morning Andrew and I found some old letters written to Mam in her youth. I took a handful of them out of their envelopes but they're all in French and the old-fashioned florid handwriting makes it pointless for me to even attempt to translate them.

'But I'm desperate to know what they say. These letters hold the answers to what happened to Mam in her teens.'

'So how can I help?' Elspeth is looking puzzled.

'I was wondering if you have a forwarding address for Adjavella?'

'I do. I'll have to check with her first of course, but I know that she'll say yes. I'll send her a text.' Elspeth reaches for her phone.

'Now comes the cheeky bit.' I say hesitantly. 'I'm terrified of parting with the originals, even though I can't read them. They are my only link to Mam's past. Is there any chance I could photocopy the letters so that I can post the copies to Adjavella? I can put some money in the petty cash to cover it.'

Elspeth smiles at me indulgently.

'That would be fine. Pass them over and I'll do it for you. Our machine is a bit temperamental. It needs an experienced hand.'

I find that handing over the precious letters, even for a moment, is surprisingly difficult. I feel the same way that I did, clutching to the hem of my mother's orange jumper dress as a child. I don't want to let go, as I am afraid to risk losing our connection.

As Elspeth settles into her rhythm with the envelopes and the letters, I fill her in on what I have uncovered in France.

It's hard to say goodbye to Elspeth, but I can't stay longer as I'm going to be late. I have a train to catch. I promise to phone before my next visit and make a proper time to catch up. She has placed all the photocopies in a large envelope and offered to post it for me, once she hears back from Adjavella. I tuck the originals safely back in my handbag, and clasping it protectively under my arm, I run to the station.

I haven't been up into the hills above Arrochar for many years. In fact, the last time that I was here, I was sixteen. We had driven up in Da's work van, the three of us sitting abreast in the cab, with all our belongings in the back.

Mam had made him scrub the van three times with a big bristle brush before she'd agreed that it was clean enough for us to use, and no longer smelled of fish.

Times had been hard financially for much of my childhood, but my parents had always protected me from it. Now, thanks to my workaholic lifestyle, I have saved more money than I could ever need. I just wish that they had let me share it with them.

However, my parents were proud and independent. The only concession that Da ever made was to let me pay the expenses related to Mam's care. He wouldn't take anything for himself.

My grief at this thought momentarily overwhelms me.

I'm heading for the campsite at Ardgartan, which had been our makeshift home during our last stay. I had a one-person tent with a li-lo, that regularly had to be topped up using the foot pump, and Ma and Da had the double mattress from their bed at home, laid out in the back of the van.

The fish van attracted a few strange looks, but I also saw several people taking down the company details. If the transport had been my choice, it would have been a deliberate marketing strategy, but Da wasn't so calculating. Our family had needed a holiday, and the van had provided the affordable solution.

We weren't the only ones using unusual transport. The Scots are an inventive bunch, and amongst the motorhomes and caravans, there were also horseboxes and flatbed farm vehicles with tarpaulins, motorcycles with flagpoles and shop awnings. You name it. If it would keep off the rain, someone was sleeping under it.

I'm so pleased that I've come back here. I'd not thought about that holiday in years. We started that trip with the forest tracks that I'm walking on today, in the foothills of The Cobbler. By the end of the week, we had climbed all the peaks in the area.

I can feel Mam and Da. It's as if they are right here beside me as I walk. Somehow, I managed to forget how comfortable I was walking with them, in my youth. Each one of us, was able to keep pace with the other two. Sometimes though I would deliberately lag behind or stride on ahead, as I knew that my parents still liked to hold hands as they enjoyed the spring of a flat grassy path under foot or whilst descending a steep stony track.

James - 1979

James is lying on his back looking at the roof of the van. He knows that he needs to broach this subject with his wife - there will be too many consequences if he doesn't - but she is not going to want to listen.

His arm is tucked under Tilly's neck, and his hand as it rests on her chest, is moving gently up and down with every breath that she takes. She is so relaxed and peaceful resting here beside him.

His next words are going to plunge her into a world of distress and pain. How can he do it to her? But Isla is asleep, and this will be the only chance that they have to talk, before the school forms have to be submitted.

'Tilly?'

'Mm?'

'We need to let Isla choose her own path.'

Tilly sits bolt upright, flinging his hand from her, and turning accusingly towards him.

'You know what they did! How can you let her study their language, their culture? She's even talking about going there! She won't be safe!'

James steels himself. When he first met Tilly, he'd had no idea of the depth of the trauma that she carried. After his first experience, he had hoped that it would fade with time, but the truth was, when triggered, her responses were just as raw and irrational as the day he first encountered them.

Most of the time, he did his best to help her avoid flashbacks to her earlier life, but occasionally, like this evening, he himself would be responsible for broaching a subject that he knew she would find disturbing. Then it was a matter of keeping Tilly safe from herself and trying not to terrify their daughter.

He speaks in hushed tones, in order not to escalate things more than necessary.

'Tilly, this is 1979. The Nazis are no longer in power. Helmut Schmidt is committed to European cooperation and to working with Britain and America within NATO. If Isla does go there, she will be safe.'

'You can't know that!' Tilly says, pulling the blankets up around her, so that James is left isolated in the centre of the mattress, in just his pyjamas. It is a freezing April night, but James is not going to be distracted.

'This decision is not even about whether Isla is safe, if she ever visits Germany. It's about whether we are going to encourage our daughter to be herself. To follow her own dreams, and to trust her own judgment. Or whether we're going to try and limit her life choices, force her to submit to our views …'

'You mean mine.'

'Well, in this instance, yes, I do. It's the principle that I am trying to protect. I believe that every person should be able to choose their own path. We both did after all, and you know how much we both hated it when our families tried to tell us what to do. That's why I am reminding you now, that when Isla was born, we promised that we would never do the same to her.'

'How can you bring that up now? That's not fair!'

'Tilly, I bring it up now, because this is the moment we were talking about. This is the time, when we have to trust her to know her own mind and do our best to support her. If you want to tell her about Camille, then you have a good chance of persuading her not to choose German, as she will know what torment it causes you.'

'Absolutely not! She must never be touched by that pain!'

'I respect your decision. But you can't then blame Isla for not understanding!'

James watches as Tilly's head sinks to rest on her knees, and the arms encircling her bent legs, hug tighter and tighter, as if she is trying to disappear into a little ball. She rocks backwards and forwards in place. The motion accelerates, faster and faster.

And here they are once again. His wife is gone, and the Tilly before him is six years old, grieving the loss of her mother. James brings his legs back underneath himself, so that he can sit up on his knees. Reaching forwards, he places his arms around his wife, and pulls her huddled form towards him.

'You are safe,' he whispers into her ear. 'You are safe, and Isla is safe,' he rubs her back gently, 'and I will not mention it again. Whatever you decide, I will support you.'

Isla -2018

I'm sitting in the car park at work, my hands still clutching the steering wheel. I need one more moment, to be certain that this is the right move. A steady stream of people in suits file past in front of my vehicle.

This has been my life for three decades. Am I sure that I can give it up?

I can feel the familiar nausea building in my stomach, and the adrenaline is causing my hands to tremble slightly as they grip the wheel.

Having felt utterly disengaged from thoughts of my future for so many weeks it now turns out, that I'm facing one of the biggest decisions I've ever made. The choices contrast so starkly from one another, and I only have ten minutes left on the clock.

Whether the decision came from an insatiable curiosity about my mother's past; the insidious anxiety that I don't know who I am either; or even the erratic behaviour that comes with grief. The astonishingly uncharacteristic decision has been made. Today I begin the first day of my retirement.

Peter and I have agreed that this is the best course of action. If I decide to return once I have found my answers, then I will do so as a consultant, as my replacement starts on Monday.

I am deeply grateful to Peter for his alternative proposal, and I'm immensely lucky that HR have been willing to keep a door open. I know that he is disappointed that I didn't want to apply for the job as his deputy, but he understands. Which is more than I can say for the part of me that fought so hard for my place in this male dominated, fast moving industry.

That part of me is furious that I'm leaving. But the truth is, I'm not the same person anymore, and thanks to Andrew and Adjavella, I have a new avenue to explore in search of my origins. Adjavella has already translated one of the letters, and more will follow shortly.

Nineteen

Isla - 2018

The physical journey has been straight forward, a train to Dusseldorf and a plane to Rennes, with a stop in Amsterdam, all at a civilised time of day, but I'm drained, exhausted, and overwhelmed.

I picked up the hire car half an hour ago, but I'm still sitting in the airport car park. The closer I get to this next phase of Mam's life, the more anxious I feel about what I must do, and what I have done. Why did I leave my fantastic job to head off on this crazy hunt?

I need to get going. There's still a two-hour journey ahead of me and I want to arrive before dark. I found an address on letters from somebody called Simone. Her surname is indecipherable in the loopy handwriting, but starts Le B. This woman wrote to my mother for a while after her arrival in Scotland.

I looked up the address on street view, so I have some chance of recognising the village and the house when I get there. Adjavella has translated one of her letters so far. From the way that she writes, it sounds like she was older than Mam. This makes the chances of her still being alive very slim, as she would be in her late eighties or more.

I'm therefore expecting to have to knock on doors searching for people that knew her. I'm not sure that my bad French is up to it. It feels so shameful that I know nothing about Mam's life in Brittany.

I can feel my defences rising against the judgments that will surely come from people unaware of Mam's secrecy. If the locals do know anything about Mam's past, will they even share it with me? They might not believe my story. I was so lucky, meeting Lis and Lorna.

I wish I'd thought to ask Lorna or Adjavella to come with me. I could have paid for Adjavella to have some time off work.

These thoughts are escalating out of control, and I'm heading for a panic attack here in the car park. I hold the steering wheel firmly between my hands and take several slow, deep breaths. Eventually it is safe to put the car in gear.

For some time now I have been travelling through another wide flat landscape. This time the roads are regularly edged with white, two-storey cottages, and terraced houses with grey, slate roofs.

Then, with one roundabout, everything changes. A vast sky opens up before me and the sandy-muddy-soup of the Baie de Plouharnel at low tide, stretches off into the distance on my left-hand side.

The railway line appears on my right - as if making another lane on the highway - but almost at once both the bay and the tracks are hidden, as I enter an avenue of trees.

The trees disappear, to be replaced by houses, as I arrive in Penthièvre. But the land is gone as well. All except the strip on which the road and the railway track have been built. It can't be more than twenty-five metres wide.

Ahead of me to the right are wartime fortifications, that according to the signs, are still owned by the Ministry of Defence. I'm glad Mam wasn't living here during the war. There would have been nowhere to run, except into the sea! It must have been very frightening.

The moment that I cross the isthmus the views of the water vanish. Historically small villages, now blend seamlessly into one another, in uncontrolled urban sprawl.

My hotel is at the farthest end of the Quiberon peninsula. It has its own car park - an important consideration in such a built-up area during peak season - and an indoor pool and spa. After all, this *is* my first week without a job in over thirty years. Even if I have no luck with my search, I intend to enjoy myself.

In honour of my new retired status, I allow myself a relaxed start to the day with coffee and a croissant in bed, curtesy of room service, before jumping into my hire car and setting the satnav for the village of Kervihan. From the map it seems to be in the central western portion of the peninsula.

The holiday traffic on the main road through the centre of the peninsula, which I drove down so freely last night, has come to a standstill. So, the satnav re-routes me diagonally across the peninsula, along smaller side streets, full of identical little white houses all with slate grey roofs.

My surroundings change as I drive into the village of Kerné. Amongst the newer structures there are several old houses, and collections of buildings that were obviously farms before the land was developed for residential use. It makes me think of my great-grandparents, and the encroaching urbanisation in Barantan.

Before I know it, the houses disappear, and are replaced by shrubby-hedgerows and rather unpromising looking fields. This pattern is repeated as I drive through several more villages. I try to strip away the newer buildings in my minds-eye, to imagine what it would have been like with just a few old farm buildings clustered at points of intersection along the narrow country lanes.

Sunny, summer days like today are deceptive. I think it would have been quite a harsh and isolated existence for Mam, living here in the 1950s. Obviously we experienced bad weather in Scotland, when I was growing up, but the area of Seamill and West Kilbride is sheltered to some degree by the Isle of Arran.

Here in Brittany, there is nothing to protect this stretch of coastline and the narrow peninsula beyond, from the full force of the waves and wind, sweeping across the Atlantic.

I take another turn towards the well-named *Côte Sauvage* or *Savage Coast* and enter the tiny village of Kervihan. Here there are many well-cared-for houses but, to my dismay, others have become complete ruins.

I feel both sadness and a sense of expectation. Here at last are some physical signs of my mother's history, a connection to the world in which she lived. Stone-walled farmhouses and lean-to sheds, slate roofs covered in lichen and moss, windows with wooden shutters and peeling paint, climbing plants that have been left undisturbed long enough in some places to reach the chimney pots. Each one adds a piece to the puzzle that was my mother's life.

I pass one old ruin where the roof is missing, and the top of a tree can be seen appearing over the front wall, from the inside of the house. I wonder if that roof was gone even when Mam lived here.

I've not been listening, and the satnav suddenly gets very excited. I've overshot my destination, and the house I'm after is back down the road a little. I turn slowly, trying to imagine the 1950s. At that time this whole area would have been just a rural hamlet, without any of the tourist chalets and holiday homes.

Holding Simone's letter in my hand, I approach the property, with a feeling of trepidation. The front garden of this former farmhouse is full of bright flowers.

A couple of climbing roses surround the door - just like at my parents' house. There is no sign of the neglect visible in some of the other old buildings in the area. These wooden shutters must have had a new lick, of the traditional blue paint, at the start of the year. … I think I've stopped breathing. … I knock and step back into the road, as if I might make a run for it.

The delay seems like minutes, but it is probably seconds before a smartly dressed woman opens the door. She is beyond retirement age. Her long, probably dyed, brown hair is swept back in a neat bun.

I summon up my best French.

'Good morning, I'm sorry to interrupt your day. I am trying to trace someone who knew a previous occupant of this house. All I know is that her first name is Simone, I believe she once knew my mother.'

The woman looks a little shocked.

'I'm sorry I don't understand, Simone Le Besco is your mother?'

'No, no!' I hurry to correct her. 'I have letters written to my mother from this address, by Simone.' I glance down at the envelope that I'm holding. 'I couldn't read the handwriting but now I see, yes her last name is Le Besco.'

'Ah! And you wish to find her.'

'Well, she would be very old now, if she were still alive, so perhaps a relative is more likely.'

'Well, you are in luck. I am her daughter, Odile.'

'You are? Oh, how nice to meet you!' I reach out my hand, and she shakes it.

'My French is not so good but from this letter I believe our mothers were great friends before Mam left the area.' I proffer the aged envelope so that she can see I am telling the truth. 'Your mother wrote very fondly to Mam.' I continue.

'What was your mother's name, maybe I knew her too?' Odile asks, ushering me through her open front door into a stone-flagged reception area.

'Tilly, Tilly MacLeod. Oh, actually when she was here, she would have been Clothilde Marec.'

There is a clatter as Odile stumbles into the side-table next to her, knocking a small wooden statue to the floor. She turns to me in astonishment.

'Your mother was Clothilde Marec? But she was my cousin.' Odile is so excited she is talking nineteen-to-the-dozen, and I can barely keep up with her French. 'Her father, and my mother, were siblings! Which makes us family!'

Odile steps forward and hugs me fiercely. I'm a little stunned and, unused to this level of physical contact, I find it hard to hug back quite so tightly. Sensing this she lets me go.

'Please, come with me to the kitchen, I'll make us some coffee. We have so much to talk about.'

I follow her down the corridor, looking carefully around me as I go. If this is my cousin, then Mam must have been here, maybe even lived, right here in this house.

'So, this was your family home, how lovely that you're still here.' I feel a sudden sadness at what I'm saying. 'I've just had to sell the house that I grew up in, as both my parents died quite soon after each other.'

'Ah, Clothilde is dead and your father too. I'm very sorry to hear that. You are right, a house holds so many memories. I found I was swamped with them, when I moved back to the area. I returned to this house a few years ago after I retired. I made the move partly to look after mother, but eventually she was unable to manage our stairs, so she moved in with my cousin Bernard and his son Philippe, down near the harbour.'

All these relatives! My head is spinning, and Odile's narrative is showing no signs of slowing down.

'That change wasn't ideal, as neither of them could cook! With two men in charge, the house got into an appalling state, but they struggled on for a while. I went every day to cook an evening meal.'

Odile fills the kettle without pausing in her tale.

'Bernard sadly died in 2015, so Philippe and I had to think again, and now there is a housekeeper that comes in regularly. It's still better than mother being here, as she has her own room on the ground floor with a bathroom next door.'

'Wait a moment, Simone is still alive? This is wonderful!'

Now it's my turn, I can barely prevent myself leaping up and hugging Odile. I don't know how I missed that Simone is still alive. My French obviously has a long way to go. If she is Odile's mother, she must be at least in her nineties by now.

I can barely sit still. I'm longing to meet her, to hear more about Mam as a young woman. Nice as it is to meet Odile, she is definitely too young to remember many details about Mam. My mind is racing ahead to our potential meeting, until a horrible thought strikes me. What if Simone also has dementia?

'Do you think she will still remember my mother?' I ask tentatively.

'Oh yes, very much so,' Odile confirms to my relief, as she places two cups of coffee on the table. 'Although she doesn't like surprises, as she has a heart condition. I'm so glad that it was me that opened the door to you today.'

The image of turning up and killing my great-aunt passes through my mind, and I am equally grateful for the way that things have turned out.

'I usually pop in to see her at lunchtime. I will break the news gently that you have come to see us, then perhaps you could join us at her house for dinner tonight.'

'That would be marvellous! Thank you. I'm so excited to meet her.'

Clothilde - 1951

The platform at Saint-Pierre Quiberon is surprisingly full. In her imagination, Clothilde had pictured herself and her aunt as the only two people at the station, so that they would have no difficulty finding each other.

Clutching her mother's precious suitcase, Clothilde heads for the luggage van to look for her trunk. She hopes that someone has remembered to off load it, as the whistle is blowing, and the train is about to leave. At least it's not far to the end of the line if it goes missing.

To her relief, her heavy wooden trunk is indeed sitting on the platform, but there is no porter to be seen, and there is no chance that she can lift it alone. In the end she takes a seat on top of it.

What she would really like to do is climb inside and let the rest of the world slip away. She's missing the farm, and Olivier immensely. Despite her best efforts to telepathically will him to ask her to stay, it didn't happen. She had been hoping that they could be married and create a life together in Barantan - given that the Stewarts had decided to abandon her.

On her last morning as she was leaving the farm, Olivier had kissed her, but it had only been the standard farewell, not the personal goodbye full of passion that she had hoped for.

Thoughts of that farewell are starting to stir memories of her final moments with the Stewarts, and she can't risk that. It's too painful. She's here in Brittany now. She must be brave. There are new relatives to meet, and a new life to begin.

The porter has returned, but the platform is now empty, except for Clothilde. He looks her way expectantly, but she shakes her head, and he walks past towards his office.

She has come all this way, and there is no one here to meet her. Despite the sunshine, it is April, and there is a cold wind blowing.

Clothilde reaches into the suitcase for her scarf. Chloe knitted it for her at Christmas. She wraps it tightly around her neck. It's lamb's wool. The softness, and the memory of the day it was given to her, makes her want to cry.

However, the moment is broken by the sound of running feet. A tall woman, with strands of mousey brown hair falling from a long plait, is hurrying towards her.

'Clothilde, is that you? I'm so sorry. Odile threw up all over me, and I had to change before I could come out.'

This must be a relative, but Clothilde is unsure whether this is her aunt Renée or her aunt Simone, and nobody mentioned Odile, perhaps it's her dog. She smiles, rising from her trunk and holding out a hand in greeting. However, her aunt has other ideas, and pulls her into a hug, kissing her warmly on both cheeks as she releases her.

The porter appears with a trolley and follows them as they walk towards the exit. Clothilde stops in her tracks. This is not what she expected to see. Outside the station, tied to the railings, is not a dog, but a horse, and the horse is between the shafts of a farm cart.

The porter has made his way to the back and is hoisting up her trunk with the assistance of her aunt, who is obviously very strong, and totally at home with such tasks.

Clothilde feels a lightness in her system that has been absent since she knew that she was moving. Her aunt lives on a farm! It won't be so different after all, and she seems nice.

Clothilde throws her suitcase and satchel up beside the trunk, and walks around to the far side, so that she can climb up beside this woman, who has so confidently taken the reigns. How can she ask her name? It seems so rude not to know.

As she lowers herself into her seat, her aunt turns to her, and with a glance over her shoulder says

'Clothilde, meet your cousin Odile.'

Clothilde flicks her head around, and there, lying nestled in a large pile of horse blankets, is a sleeping child. She must be about six months old and is making small sucking movements with her mouth as she sleeps.

'Is she your daughter?' Clothilde asks, somewhat unnecessarily.

'Yes, she was born in October last year. I'm afraid that's the reason Neven and I can't invite you to live at the farm with us'

They can't! Clothilde stops breathing. Where is she going to live? She'd already planned her whole future in her head. Her aunt was going to think her such an asset for knowing farming life inside out. They would become friends, and she would fit in.

But none of that is going to happen.

Her aunt continues to speak, as she encourages the horse to walk out onto the road, unaware of the distress that her words have caused her niece.

'Renée and Jagu are in a far better position to take you in. Bernard is almost ten years old, and they have a much bigger house. Also, you will be closer to your school, and to the other children, should you want to meet them at the beach.'

Clothilde bristles at the word children. She hasn't thought of herself as a child for many years. For goodness sake, she will be fifteen next month, and old enough to marry Olivier, if only he had asked her.

'I remember what it was like being fourteen,' her aunt continues. 'I wanted to be with my friends all the time.'

'But I don't have any friends!' Clothilde mutters under her breath.

They travel along the main road a short way, and then turn right onto a smaller lane.

'I'm going to take you back to our farm for a while until Renée and her family return home. The farm's at Kervihan, which is in the middle of the peninsula. The grazing is better away from the coast, but it's only a ten-minute walk to the beach on the Atlantic side. Of course, if you want to swim, it will take you about half an hour to walk to Drehen.'

'I've never swum in the sea before,' Clothilde confesses. 'We only had the river, and I didn't really swim.'

'Well, we'll have to teach you.' Simone replies enthusiastically. 'The water's pretty cold right now, but it will warm up soon enough.'

Unsure what to say next, Clothilde looks ahead of her, between the ears of the horse. Just as in Barantan, there are a lot of new houses being built on the farmland beside the lane, and during their short journey, they have already been overtaken by several cars.

Isla - 2018

In order to see some more of the area where Mam grew up, I take the alternative route back along the Atlantic coast road. There's no development here at all, probably because of the buffeting that houses would receive, from the prevailing winds and winter storms.

The high cliffs are punctuated by a series of tiny coves. A few of these are currently host to some intrepid surfers, their black wetsuits only visible against the dark swirl of the waves because they are framed by the stark white edges of their boards.

As I near the tip of the peninsula, multiple tourists can be seen, searching for the small collection of standing stones that are scattered around the beginning of the Côte Sauvage.

I read about these in the guidebook, and was expecting something like Stonehenge in the UK, or the French standing stones at Carnac - that I believe are impressive, although I've only seen a photograph.

However, these ones are so spread out, and small, that without the guidebook, I would never have realised that they were anything other than part of the natural landscape.

Odile told me that Simone and Philippe live in one of the streets off to the left here, but the address is in my handbag in the boot of the car, and I'm keen to head back to the hotel. I will see where they are soon enough.

The traffic is stop-start as I weave my way through the crowds of shoppers, and up through the central tourist zone. In this area it is impossible to strip away the twenty-first century. Not a single old cottage is left. The modern apartments and hotels are interspersed with parades of shops and more industrial buildings. The farmland in this section is completely gone.

Twenty

Isla - 2018

Back at the hotel I take a piece of headed paper from the desk drawer and turn it over to use the blank side. I'm getting so confused by all these new family members. For most of my life it has been so straight forward - just Mam, Da, and me.

With each conversation I have, I'm forced to dismantle my understanding of the world, and re-form it according to a new pattern. Each new relative that I meet adds their own thread to the story, which must be carefully woven into the fabric according to the new blueprint.

I am struck by the way that this process is the absolute inverse of Mam's mental decline. For her the fully woven, vibrant fabric of her life history gradually unravelled one memory, one person at a time, until we were all gone. The deep sorrow that floods me, so acutely, at this thought takes several minutes to subside.

As I collect up the soggy tissues that have amassed on the desk, I experience the familiar niggle at the back of my mind. Is this need to write it all down normal? Surely, in years gone by, I would have been able to keep this new information straight in my mind, without the need for a chart. … I never did make that appointment with my GP.

Whatever the truth of this, I still need to draw a family tree. As Henri has brought me to Quiberon, I start with him. Turning the paper to landscape, I write my grandfather's name, Henri Marec, about four centimetres down on the left-hand side of the page, leaving room in case I discover any ancestors older than him. Then I add his wife Camille, Mam, Da, and me. Easy.

I've decided not to place Camille's Barantan family on this chart, as it will only confuse things.

Next, in the middle of the page, and at the same level as Mam, I add Odile, and across from her on the right-hand side, Bernard, followed by his death date, 2015.

Clothilde, Odile, and Bernard are three first-cousins. It's nice to think of them growing up here together.

Under Bernard, and level with me, I then add Philippe - his son, and my second cousin - who is still alive.

I don't think Philippe has a family of his own, as Odile didn't mention children or a partner being part of the household, so I return upwards to add Simone, above Odile, in line with Henri.

There are gaps, for example I don't know anything about Bernard's parents, but at least I should be able to keep these people straight in my mind.

It's a nice evening so I decide to leave the car in the hotel car park and walk to Simone's. I have plenty of time, so I head down to join the coast road at the Plage du Goviro.

This beach, at the foot of the peninsula, faces due south. It's a clear day, and in the distance, I catch a glimpse of the island Belle-Île-en-mer across the water.

I've been told it's a beautiful place for a day trip by ferry, but I'm not sure that I'll be doing any sightseeing whilst I'm here. I turn right and head towards the town's main beach.

I'm passed by a string of young families all carrying buckets and spades, and bags of groceries. They are heading for the camping grounds that are tucked in amongst the trees behind me.

Despite this, La Grande Plage is far from empty. The tide is on its way in, but there is still plenty of sand for the older tourists waiting for the bars to open, and the shop assistants trying to catch a little sunshine after work.

At the far end of the bay, I pause to make a small detour out onto the jetty at Port Maria. In my mother's day, before major mechanisation, this would have been a thriving fishing port. Now, most of the boats in the harbour are privately owned pleasure boats.

I rest my elbows on the harbour wall and look west, towards the Atlantic. Strangely, there's a castle on the next headland that looks as if it's been dropped from a fairy tale. It has an odd mixture of towers and turrets, and looks ready for Rapunzel, or some other damsel to be rescued from capture and confinement in the castle at Land's End.

I retrace my steps and head inland towards Kervozès and Manémeur. At one time these would have been two separate hamlets, but now housing is continuous across the lower end of the peninsula.

I catch sight of Philippe's house. Unlike many adjacent homes, this one has beautiful thick farmhouse walls, and a well-kept yet weathered appearance that speaks of generations of occupation.

Clothilde - 1951

Clothilde opens her eyes and stares at the ceiling. The air feels damp and smells different. It's probably the salt from the sea. She caught a glimpse of the ocean from the train yesterday as they crossed the isthmus onto the peninsula, but she can't wait for her first ever visit to a beach.

Her new room is tucked in under the eaves and very small. There's just enough space for a single bed, a chest of drawers and very soon her trunk. It's still on the cart up at the farm, but Uncle Neven is going to bring it tonight and help carry it up the stairs.

There's no ceiling height for a wardrobe, but this tiny room suits her perfectly. Her aunt and uncle won't be able to ask her to share with anyone else. All she wants right now is some privacy to grieve.

However, she can hear people moving around downstairs, so she'd better rise and see if she can be useful. She must earn her keep after all.

Clothilde throws back the covers and steps out onto the sheepskin that is covering the floorboards beside her bed. She kneels on it, so that she can reach under the bed for the big suitcase that she stored safely there on her arrival.

Pulling it out, she raises the lid so that she can view the few personal items that she owns. Two beautiful dresses made for her last year by her grandmother. She lifts them carefully, and places them on the bed. The folder of documents - that prove who she is, and the schools that she has attended - follows.

What she seeks is underneath. The tiny suitcase that she herself carried all the way from Paris to Barantan when she was a little girl. It is filled with the most precious items of all.

It still holds the children's book and the bear that made that journey with her, but now in place of her infant clothing, there are two dictionaries. The first, in French, was given to her by her grandfather in 1946 to help with her schoolwork.

The second, in English, had only been given to her last week by Rory. He said that he was concerned that she might not keep up her second language, as she would no longer be speaking it on a regular basis. Whose fault is that?

Although she's sure that one day she'll be glad to have it, right now she's so angry with him, that all she wants to do is throw it out of the window.

The gift that she's after this morning is from Lorna. Lorna told her not to open it until she arrived at her destination. So now, it's time to see what her friend has given her.

For the first week, after hearing Rory's decision, Clothilde had been just as cross with Lorna, as with her parents, but now she is trying to be more reasonable. After all, it's not Lorna's fault that they're moving, and her friend was always going to leave Barantan for teaching college.

Clothilde pulls out the little cloth pouch, and leaning back against the bed frame, tips the contents into her hand. There is a folded piece of paper, some money, and a little packet inscribed with the words: *To wear whenever you need a friend.* Clothilde unwraps it and discovers four beautiful hairclips decorated with roses.

Lorna knows her so well. She has protected Clothilde from loneliness every day since she was five years old and is still trying to do the same with this gift, despite their separation.

Clothilde swallows hard. How will she face every day without the girl, who in all respects except blood, was a big sister, and yet better, because she was a companion and confidant, but never a rival.

The fact that these clips are decorated with roses, Clothilde's symbol of love, is not an accident.

Lorna helped her care for the rose bush in the vegetable garden, planted all those years ago in memory of Henri. She was also there when the village planted the ones along the barn wall for Camille after her disappearance.

When Joseph died, Lorna bought Chloe and Clothilde a beautiful climbing rose for the doorway of the farmhouse, and she knows, that on coming here, Clothilde has had to leave all of these precious plants behind.

Clothilde picks up the folded paper. It is a note from Lorna.

This money is so that you can by more rose bushes, for Chloe and the rest of the family. When we move, I will try and give the other plants a new home in Le Vernet, so that one day you can visit them again.

The tears well in Clothilde's eyes. This is the most overwhelming gift.

Isla - 2018

I can feel the nerves building inside me at the thought of meeting Simone. I knock on the door and am pleased that it's Odile who answers.

'Isla, welcome, come in, mother is in the front room. Come and join us for a drink.'

She continues to talk as I follow her into a room full of old dark-wood furniture. Several pieces have beautifully upholstered seats and I wonder if they are the handiwork of Simone's sister.

'Unfortunately, Philippe already had dinner plans tonight, so he is unable to join us, but he hopes that you can visit again, perhaps some time over the weekend. He definitely wants to meet you before you have to leave.'

Although I'm sad not to meet Philippe, it is Simone that I am desperate to see. She's sitting in an upright chair, to the side of a high, round coffee table. Probably to avoid difficulties rising, from what is otherwise low furniture in the rest of the room. I approach as Odile introduces me.

'Maman, this is Isla, Clothilde's daughter.'

'I'm so delighted to meet you.' I say as I bend down and offer her my hand. 'Thank you for having me to dinner.'

Simone sits up straight in her chair. She is surprisingly tall, and although she has the thinness of extreme old age, I can see that once she was broad-shouldered and athletic. She peers at me through a milky white film that I can see obscuring her vision.

'Come closer my dear. I want to see if you smell like her.'

Slightly startled. I step closer.

'I don't think I do. I probably smell more of shower gel and perfume, but it's a nice idea.'

When she has sniffed me without comment, I take a seat in the chair on the other side of the little table, so that she can at least see an impression of me as we talk.

'We are drinking sherry. It's mother's favourite.' Odile says as she crosses the room to a tray with glasses and a crystal decanter. 'Would you like some, or can I offer you something else?'

'Sherry would be lovely.' I reply, unable to think of the last time I drank a glass.

'Where are you staying?' Simone asks.

'In a hotel near the aerodrome. It's very comfortable.'

'Have you seen much of the area yet?' Simone continues, in what feels a little like an interrogation, but perhaps she's as nervous as I am.

'I'm biased, but I love it here. I never understood why Clothilde wanted to move away.'

And there it is, the thorny issue that is so hard to explain. I side-step having to comment by focusing on her question.

'I've not done much exploring yet, although on my way here I walked past that fairy tale castle on the headland. It seems so out of character with the area. More like something we would have in Germany.'

'That's Le Chateau Turpault' Odile supplies. 'It was built in 1904 by a wealthy businessman. It's a private residence and none of us have ever been inside.'

'You said *like we would have in Germany*, do you live there?' Simone asks in a quavering voice.

I can't believe my carelessness. I was trying so hard not to mention Mam leaving that I forgot to avoid mentioning where I live. I'd been so determined to avoid conflict today. Especially with Simone and her heart condition.

My experience with Mam has taught me that people who lived through the Second World War don't necessarily share my positive view of modern Germany. I take a deep breath and begin.

'I moved to Germany thirty years ago. It caused great conflict with Mam, which I have only come to understand in recent months. I'm sorry if where I've made my home upsets you as much as it did her.'

I reach out across the table and place my hand over Simone's narrow wrinkled one. She covers it with her other one and squeezes mine to reassure me.

'Clothilde suffered huge loss because of the Nazi invasion of France. She was much more personally affected than we were. Yes, Henri was my brother, and his death in the bombing raid on the railway depot was a devastating blow to our family, but it was wartime, and adults understand that death and loss are a huge part of war. Most families in France were touched in one way or another.'

'Mam was a complicated person.' I try to explain. 'In fact, I only discovered that she was French last November.'

There is a stunned silence in the room.

'You didn't know that your mother was French? How is that possible?' Simone asks.

'She spoke English with a beautiful Scottish accent, and short of saying that her parents died when she was very young, she never spoke about her past.'

'But James, your father, did he never mention Quiberon to you?' Odile shakes her head in puzzlement.

'Why would he? … Wait! … How do you know that my father was called James?'

'Because this is where your parents met!'

I stare at Simone in astonishment.

Twenty-one

Clothilde - 1956

Clothilde is with Simone at the farm when Bernard comes to find her.

'Clothilde, they need your help at the doctor's house.' He pants, resting his hands on his knees to catch his breath.

'My help? What can I do? I'm not a nurse.' She replies grumpily.

'It's not for nursing, they need a translator.'

Clothilde still doesn't understand and hasn't moved. Bernard is infuriated and grabs her hand, pulling her towards his bicycle.

'The man is really hurt, and they can't understand him. The doctor thinks he might be Scottish. Lorna's father was Scottish, wasn't he?'

Bernard looks at his cousin expectantly.

'I told them that he taught you his language. I'm sure you're going to understand him.'

Bernard is looking ridiculously proud of himself. He obviously thinks this is a chance to prove that he can be useful to the men. He has complained a lot recently about them treating him as a child, and he wants nothing more than to secure a job for the summer on one of the boats.

Intrigued, Clothilde darts forward, and grabs the bike from where it's leaning up against the wall. She jumps on it, shouting.

'I'm in front, you'll have to ride on the back.' Then without waiting, she stands up on the pedals and sets off down the lane, with Bernard chasing behind.

Clothilde's bravura diminishes as she approaches the building, and by the time she reaches the surgery, she is following several steps behind Bernard.

What if this man isn't Scottish? What if he is, but she can't understand him? It's now more than five years since she spoke English to anyone. If she fails, everyone will think she's dumb. The teasing over her Auvergne accent has only recently stopped, now that she's no longer in school, and she's not certain she wants to open up the possibility of ridicule from the adults, when they hear her speaking English.

'Ah! Wonderful. Bernard, you found your cousin!' Dr Aubuchon booms as he spots them at the end of the corridor. 'Come, follow me!'

Clothilde does as she's told and is soon standing at the foot of a hospital bed containing a very handsome young man. She's not quite sure where to look, as he is not wearing many clothes. His chest is bare, and his left arm is supported across his chest in a sling.

A nurse is currently examining his cheekbones for signs of damage, as he has two purple, black eyes. His other hand is bandaged, and they are organising a hoist for his left leg, which is obviously badly broken.

'What on Earth happened?' Clothilde asks.

She had intended to speak to the doctor, but because her thoughts switched language on the cycle ride, it came out in English.

'I had an accident on the trawler.'

Clothilde's eyes flick up and fix on the young man. He's definitely Scottish, but the accent's not quite the same as Rory's.

She smiles and steps closer.

'My name's Clothilde. They want to know how you're feeling.'

'Nice to meet you, Clothilde. I'm James. James MacLeod. I'd shake your hand, but I don't think that's going to be possible for a while.'

He smiles wryly, shrugging his shoulders and yelping in pain as his broken collar bone shifts.

'Don't move please!' She urges him, with a panicked look on her face. She casts her eyes towards the doctor, but he is already moving in to help.

'How are you able to understand what I say?' James asks. 'You speak English with a great Scottish accent by the way!'

James pauses because of the pain but takes a deep breath and continues.

'It's lovely, but a bit disconcerting. I've never heard of a French person with a Scottish accent before.'

Clothilde can feel herself being pulled into a vortex of emotion, that she's desperate to avoid, so she says, 'A Scotsman helped raise me,' and leaves it at that.

Dr Aubuchon has a series of questions for James about his injuries, and Clothilde passes on his explanations of the treatment that James will receive. James's relief is obvious. However, as there are several other patients next door in the waiting room the doctor leaves.

Bernard has already lost interest and gone home, so Clothilde finds herself completely alone with the stranger.

'I still don't understand how you ended up here.' she admits.

'I was working with my cousin on the trawlers off the Cornish coast, but I wanted to travel a bit more before going back to Scotland, so for the last few months I've hopped around the South coast of Britain, hiring myself out as extra crew in whichever port we landed the catch from the previous trip.'

Clothilde's feet are getting tired so, as James talks, she crosses the room to fetch an upright chair.

'This most recent boat was based in the Scilly Isles. I was intending to head back towards Newlyn the next time we went ashore, but it looks like I may have to wait a while.'

James glances down at his broken body.

'But why did they bring you all the way here when you had your accident? We don't even have a hospital.' Clothilde asks, placing the chair so that James doesn't have to twist to see her.

'On Monday we got news of a giant shoal of pilchards off the French coast. The captain was sure that we could make it there and back before the storm hit, even though none of the other boats were trying it.'

'You were out in the storm on Tuesday night?' Clothilde is appalled.

It had been one of the worst Atlantic storms she had ever experienced. The winds had ripped the roofs off several buildings across the peninsula, and many of the boats in the harbour were damaged, despite the protection of the jetty.

'We were holed up in the cabin, and doing ok, but then one of the nets broke loose. I went out on deck to try and secure it. But instead, it got whipped up by the wind and wrapped itself all around me. I tried to unravel it, but instead I got all tangled up. The wind was phenomenal. I've never known anything like it. It picked up the net with me in it, and as the boat tipped in the waves, I was slammed all over the deck.'

Without realising it, Clothilde has reached out her hand and is resting it compassionately on James's knee, where it lies beside her under the blanket.

'I have to confess I was terrified.' he continues. 'Each time I hit the deck the force was immense. One of my feet, and both my hands were tangled in the netting, and there was absolutely nothing I could do to free myself.'

'But you did manage it eventually.' Clothilde is gripped by the story and transfixed by his deep, grey-blue eyes.

'No, the others came to my rescue. They found a knife and cut the net free of its tethers on the deck, so that the whole tangled mess - with me in the middle - could be brought into the wheelhouse. One great sook threw up at the sight of my foot pointing the wrong way, and my arm all disconnected from my shoulder. It took them twenty minutes to cut me free.'

Clothilde is also feeling a little queasy at the thought of James' limbs all broken and twisted. He must have been in such pain.

'By the time they'd rescued me, we were even more off course. The only thing we could do was ride out the storm and try to stay afloat. When the sea finally calmed enough for our captain to set his own course, this part of your coast was the nearest place he could try and obtain help for me.'

'So where are the others now?' Clothilde glances towards the door to the corridor.

'They've gone.'

Clothilde can't believe what he's just said.

'It's ok,' James continues seeing her expression. 'They couldn't hang around. Every day the boat's not at sea, puts their livelihood in jeopardy. Maybe if the accident had happened to one of their friends they would have stayed, but it's not as if any of them knew me.'

'So, you're here all alone?' Clothilde squeezes his knee tightly. 'Can you speak any French at all?'

'No. I didn't plan to come here, otherwise I would have brought a phrase book at least.' James gives her a half wink and a weak smile. 'The medical staff are finding it very difficult to understand my West Coast accent, so it looks like you, Clothilde, are my only hope.'

Clothilde glows. This is going to be a chance to prove to everyone in Quiberon that her background is actually an advantage. She's also going to be able to spend lots of time with this lovely boy. For sadly, having watched him carefully whilst he's been talking, and brave and independent though he obviously is, he can only be eighteen at the most.

For several years now she's been hoping to find a man to share her life, as it's obvious to her, that a woman alone is vulnerable, both personally and financially.

However, she doesn't want just anyone, she wants someone she can rely on, someone who understands the importance of stability and security and knows that these take hard work and careful planning to achieve. A boy will not understand this, especially one who has set out to explore the world, with no responsibility to anyone except himself.

However, just because James is a couple of years younger than she is, it doesn't mean that they can't be friends. In fact, she could really do with a friend because, whilst she has formed reasonable relationships with her new family, a close friendship is something she has never quite achieved in the five years that she's been living here.

James - 1956

James looks up to see his new friend Clothilde walking through the door of the surgery. He is so thankful for her arrival. He has been lying in exactly the same spot for days, and the boredom and frustration is almost more than he can bear, even without the pain.

He relishes the way that she moves, as she follows her now familiar routine, of retrieving the upright chair and placing it in the perfect spot beside his bed. Close enough to create intimacy whilst they talk, and yet at a distance that avoids him having to twist. As she sits down, she reaches into the pocket of her overcoat and pulls out a book, which she places in his lap with a flourish.

'You've got to give me credit. I screwed up my courage and braved a visit to my former schoolteacher to borrow this.'

James squints down at the hard-backed book lying in his lap.

'I can't see.' He complains, nudging it with his free but bandaged hand.

Clothilde picks it up and turns the spine towards him.

'I'm sorry, I keep forgetting that you can't hold anything. The school library didn't have much choice for material written in English. The English literature section was tiny. This volume of Shakespeare sonnets looked the most approachable. Would you like me to read one of them aloud?'

James is unsure whether Shakespeare is really his thing, but at the sound of her voice, a smile spreads across his face, and he lies back, listening to her read.

Once again Clothilde is at James's bedside reading to him, but he can't concentrate. It's three weeks since his accident, and he is beside himself with worry. His right hand has now healed, and his broken collarbone is improving. The torn muscles around his dislocated left shoulder are also mending but his leg is another matter.

It has been badly broken in multiple places and the doctor seems concerned that he might lose it. This isn't something that he's learnt from Clothilde, and he's been glad that she's blissfully unaware of his predicament. However, he can't keep it from her any longer, as he needs her to speak to the doctor on his behalf.

Knowing that he can't speak French, the medical staff have been talking freely in front of him when she isn't around, unfortunately forgetting that a large part of human communication is body language.

In addition to the problems aligning the broken bones, one of his wounds has developed an infection and although they change the dressing regularly, he isn't sure if it's healing successfully. The thought of amputation is terrifying, but even if that doesn't happen, his plan for a future working on the trawlers will require complete physical fitness, and it's not looking good.

'Clothilde, the doctor will be here any minute. I need you to ask him something for me.'

'Of course.'

Clothilde closes the book and looks up into his face.

'It's my leg. They won't tell me if it is going to heal properly. I think that they have decided not to amputate…'

'Oh my God! Amputation! They never mentioned that to me.'

He shouldn't have put it so bluntly. She's really upset.

'I'm pretty sure it no longer looks necessary. Could you check, and also see if they can give a time frame for when I'll be able to walk again?'

'You want to go home. I understand.'

Clothilde looks sad and puts the book of sonnets on the seat behind her.

'No, that's not it at all. I want to be able to leave this place. I'm the only inpatient, and I'm totally bored - except when you are here.' he says quickly, to reassure her.

'I want to go outside with you to look at the ocean. To feel the sand between my toes and breathe fresh air. I'm an outdoor lad. I hate being cooped up all day, and I've been inside nearly a month.'

Clothilde visibly relaxes.

'Perhaps we can borrow a wheelchair and I can push you out in it.'

'I can't ask you to do that.' James is suddenly unsure of himself. 'You'd be exhausted.'

'Why? You're not so heavy, and I'm used to working on the farm. It would be fun!'

Isla - 2018

Simone has a faraway look in her eyes as she speaks. I can't believe what I'm hearing.

'Da was here?' I'm incredulous. 'He never said anything.'

'Your father had an accident at sea, and your mother was the only person who could understand his thick Scottish accent when he was brought here to the doctor. They became inseparable.'

'How old were they when this happened?'

I'm struggling to match this new information with the story my parents told me of their first meeting. It seems that, once again, my parents have given me, not exactly lies, but half-truths.

Da had always said that his boat had docked in Mam's home port. The story was that their eyes met across a crowded room, and before they knew it, they were deep in a conversation, which forged a connection that lasted them more than half a century. They just left out the part where this happened in France!

'James was very young, just eighteen. Your mother was a couple of years older. She had left school and was helping Neven and I up at the farm. We didn't have enough work for her full time, but she would come most days anyway and often spent time with Odile, teaching her to do her sums and little bits of English for fun.'

'Those sessions around the kitchen table are what I remember the best about your mother.' Odile interrupts 'I looked forward to them immensely because I got her all to myself. I was six when James arrived, and I was a bit put out because she started spending all her spare time with him, instead of with me.'

I can see the depth of her childhood feelings playing across her face as Odile relives the memory. I feel sorry for the little girl losing her playmate as romance blossomed.

'So, they were almost childhood sweethearts.'

It's quite astonishing to me that they could have been so certain of each other at such a young age.

'They kept it secret from us for several months.' Simone tips her head towards the ceiling as she settles into her memory.

'Renée disapproved of him, and both Neven and Jagu thought he was much too young to get married. I, on the other hand, liked your father. I could see how relaxed Clothilde was with him, and that was unusual for her.'

Clothilde - 1956

The wheelchair is old and bulky and, although she will only admit it to herself, much heavier than Clothilde had expected.

James appears rather self-conscious to be out in public, pushed by a girl. He's dressed in an oversized shirt and jacket borrowed from the doctor, as the clothes he was wearing when he arrived were bloody rags.

Although his duffel bag made it with him from the boat, when Clothilde unpacked it for him, it had only contained the trousers he is now wearing, some under garments, and an Arran jumper that he seems particularly attached to, although it has no useful purpose in this warm weather. Not to mention the trouble it would be to put it on over his head, as his arm is still in a sling.

They leave the Rue de Kermorvan and head out towards Port Haliguen. The streets are smooth and flat. Clothilde manages to gain enough momentum for the chair to roll along with little effort.

After fifteen minutes James is visibly thrilled to catch sight of the sea a short way ahead but becomes concerned as he feels Clothilde slowing down.

'What's the matter?' he asks, trying to turn his head to look at her.

She brings the chair to a halt and walks around so that he can see her.

'The first part of the route is so flat that I'd forgotten this last bit, from here to the harbour, is quite steep. If we go down there, I'm not sure I will be able to push you back up again.'

James's face falls. He's obviously desperate to make it to the water's edge.

Clothilde understands his disappointment, but she knows it's foolish to go ahead. Especially given that he can't possibly walk on his leg.

'It's a port, isn't it?' James is not giving up just yet. 'Are there any cafés or bars down there?'

'You can't be that desperate for a drink can you?' Clothilde is not impressed.

'No.'

James is obviously shocked that she would make that assumption but insists.

'Seriously, are there?'

'Yes.' Clothilde replies, slightly grumpily.

She's already tired from pushing and doesn't want to be bullied into a reckless decision.

'Well then, we're ok. Where there is drinking, there are men, and they will take one look at you, and come to the aid of a damsel in distress.'

Clothilde looks sceptical, so James continues.

'And if they don't like the look of me, I will pay them - as long as they take British pounds!'

Clothilde snorts with laughter.

'Ok, if you're that desperate we'll do it. I'm sure I can manage. Can you rest your good hand on the wheel to help me brake on the way down?'

James - 1956

James is sitting in his wheelchair, happily breathing in huge amounts of salty air. He glances back at the harbour and can see several groups of men sitting outside the hotel drinking beer. He is fairly certain that if Clothilde explains how he was injured, his fellow fishermen will help them back up the hill.

'You mentioned money earlier.'

Clothilde's voice, tinged with anxiety, interrupts his thoughts. She is sitting below him on the end of the jetty, dangling her feet over the edge.

'How are you going to manage? Especially as you can't work.'

'I'm ashamed to admit that I haven't given it much thought until now. The doctor hasn't mentioned anything yet, but now that I'm up and about, it's only a matter of time.'

'Have you really got some cash with you?'

'Yes, luckily my last couple of jobs were back-to-back and it wasn't possible to go ashore for any length of time, so I didn't spend any of it. But I do need to swap it into Francs. Might you be able to push me to a bank tomorrow, so that I can see if they're able to help me?'

'Of course!'

Clothilde seems to brighten at the news that he is not destitute. Hopefully, she's even a little excited at the prospect of another day out in his company.

James knows for certain that there is nothing else he would rather do.

Isla - 2018

Now that she's started talking, I'm keen to take this opportunity to mine Simone's memory for every scrap of information I can about my mother, so I start with a fairly fundamental question.

'What was Mam like as a young woman? She had been through so much before she got here. It's hard to imagine how she coped.'

For the last six months I've been trying to put myself in my mother's shoes and have found it impossible. In part, this is because I'm not the most naturally empathetic person, but also because her traumatic early life is so far from any experiences of my own. I'm finding it hard to locate parallel, relatable concepts to assist my imagination.

'When Clothilde first arrived here, she was exceedingly polite and very formal. I think she was desperate to avoid any possibility of being sent away. This lasted several months, along with a tendency to remain in her room unless she was needed.'

I recognise this excessively polite, brittle version of Mam. It would come out amongst strangers, and in any situation involving authority.

'She would go out alone on foot, mostly to the Côte Sauvage so that she could avoid contact with people, and she would return with red eyes and a puffy face, but she never cried in front of us.'

Once again this is something I recognise. As a child I would know that my mother was upset because of her absence - either behind a closed door, or from the house - rather than because she showed any form of emotion in front of me.

'It took over six months, but eventually she felt secure enough in her position here within our family to express her opinions, and at times they clashed with those of the adults around her - as is so true for any teenager - but with Clothilde, you always got a sense that she felt alone against the world in these moments, she wasn't aligning herself with her peers against the older generation.'

Odile stands and collects the empty sherry glasses.

'The dinner is almost ready. We're going to eat in the kitchen. Maman, would you like a hand?'

'No, no, I'm fine.' Simone bats away her extended arm. 'I will just make a visit to my room on the way. Isla, as we have a few minutes would you like to go up and see where your mother slept when she lived here. I can't accompany you I'm afraid, but it's easy to find. Just keep going up the stairs until they run out. Her room was under the eaves.'

I'm no longer listening properly.

'Mam lived here?' It's a good thing that I'm still sitting down, as my legs have gone to jelly. I don't know why I'm so surprised. Mam must have lived somewhere with family members, but I'd been so intent on my search for Simone. Then I met Odile and I'd assumed that Mam had lived at the house in Kervihan, and that I would have a chance for a proper look around the next time that I visited.

Simone puts me straight.

'Yes, she lived here with Renée and Jagu for almost ten years. She had the little room upstairs next to what is now the bathroom.'

I climb the stairs. I can feel my heart beating in my chest and notice that I'm holding my breath. As I push open the small wooden door it catches part way on a knotted rug that is covering the wooden floorboards.

The space is no bigger than a monk's cell, with a low window at ankle level. During the day this would let in a reasonable amount of light, but right now, it leaves the room in almost total darkness, as dusk has fallen in the outside world. A distant streetlight is all that I can see.

I feel for a light switch on the wall but there isn't one, so I take my phone from my pocket to use as a torch.

The room is truly tiny, and from what Simone has just said, Mam spent hours alone in here. A wrought iron, single bed frame with an old horsehair mattress is tucked into the corner, and next to it is a small table with a lamp. I cross the room and switch it on as I sit down on the bed.

I feel desperate for Mam. This cupboard-of-a-room is where she found herself when she left Lorna. She went from having a place in two loving households in the Auvergne, to a tiny attic room in a rather bleak house, on the edge of the Atlantic Ocean.

Simone and Odile seem to be nice people, but they have none of Lorna's natural ebullience, and anyway this wasn't even their house. From its furnishings - which I imagine from their style have been here since Renée and Jagu lived here - the house has an air of *doing things properly*.

I can imagine that the contrast with what Mam had known in Barantan would have been difficult. Especially in the first few months while she was getting to know everyone.

I kick off my shoes and lie down on the mattress. Turning onto my side, so that I can see the dark shadows of the clouds on the night sky through the tiny window. I pull the uncovered pillow down in front of my belly, and with my head resting on my folded left arm, I hug the pillow tightly with the other.

Did Mam lie like this, staring out at the new world she found herself in, unsure of her welcome, and desperate to return home?

Clothilde - 1951

Clothilde makes her way down the stairs to the kitchen. It's neat and tidy, with a much more formal feel than any of the homes she's grown up with in the Auvergne. Renée is wearing an apron, and has her dark hair tied back in a scarf. She is pouring coffee for her husband, who, already in fishing gear, is cleaning his penknife at the kitchen sink.

'Would you like to go down to the harbour with Jagu today?' Renée asks. 'He can introduce you to a few people, and you can take a look around. I will be coming down later to make some purchases, so we could meet at the café, and then go to the shops together.'

Clothilde forms the distinct impression that Renée wants her out from under her feet for a few hours whilst she cleans the house, even though it looks like it was done thoroughly yesterday before she arrived.

This is going to be a whole new way of living. A certain level of dirt was just taken for granted at the farm. There was always too much to do outside to worry about the house.

Twenty-two

Clothilde - 1951

Clothilde is relieved. She has survived her first full day here in Quiberon. Her aunt is still very reserved, but at least the fishermen this morning, were friendly. In fact, one or two of them had been a little too friendly for her liking.

However, she doubts she'll have to worry, as Jagu spotted them, and warned them off with a glare. It's nice to know that he will be looking out for her.

School starts tomorrow, and Clothilde is not looking forward to it. She's always been interested in learning, but she's never found it easy to make friends. In the past she had Lorna, so friends at school were less important.

Now she is on her own. This is a difficult time of year to join an existing group of students. Everyone will be revising for exams, and many in her year will be thinking of leaving school altogether.

Who's going to be interested in talking to the new girl?

Clothilde sits down, in what has become her favourite spot - the sheepskin on the floor by her bed. From here she can see out of the low window across the fields to the dark-grey line in the distance that is the sea.

Somehow, it comforts her to know that she is on the edge of something, at a point of transition. She's at the very edge of France. The moment where the land meets the sea, and beyond that sea is America.

She and Lorna met some American soldiers in Barantan at the end of the war. They had fallen about laughing at the idea of two little French girls with Scottish accents and had been astonished that they could chat so easily with them in English, although it had taken a while for all of them to make sense of the varying pronunciation.

Here too, Clothilde is learning that having a shared language is really no guarantee of comprehension. The people in this region speak with a very different inflection to their French, which she is finding confusing. She's frustrated that she has to repeat herself so often when she talks to her family.

Hopefully it will be better at school tomorrow, as more of her interactions will be written down. The last thing that she needs is to begin her school career looking stupid in front of the class.

Isla - 2018

I enter Philippe's kitchen to a fantastically fishy smell.

'Take a seat,' Odile gestures to the empty place opposite her mother. 'This soup is a local speciality. I hope you like it.'

'It smells delicious.' I sit as directed and I am about to follow Odile's lead and tuck in when Simone leans back in her seat and starts to laugh.

'Do you remember the night we celebrated Clothilde's arrival in Quiberon?' Simone looks across at her daughter but quickly corrects herself 'Oh no, of course you don't, wrong generation.'

I put my spoon back down, intrigued to hear what will follow.

'Renée had spent hours preparing a special meal for us all, as Neven and I were dropping by with Clothilde's trunk. You were asleep in a basket.' Simone says turning to her daughter with an indulgent look. 'Anyway, as you've done tonight, Renée's whole meal was based around local cuisine, to welcome Clothilde to the area.'

Clothilde -1951

The family is crowded around the kitchen table, which in Clothilde's honour, has been laid with the best china, and a beautiful, long floral table-decoration. She is a little embarrassed to be the centre of attention. However, she's pleased that Simone and Neven are here to help keep the conversation flowing. The shopping trip with Renée this morning was a rather silent affair.

The back door opens, and Jagu enters, with a large platter piled high with big flat shells and segments of lemon.

'Fresh from the sea - tuck in.' He says, placing the platter in the centre of the table.

Each family member reaches forward and selects a shell. Clothilde watches in horror as, one after the other, they prod the contents with the tip of a knife to check that it moves, squeeze a wedge of lemon, add a little pepper, and pop the contents straight in their mouths.

'But they're alive, how can you?' she shrieks.

'Have you never had an oyster before?' Jagu asks.

'They don't have them in the Auvergne,' Renée says, in a surprisingly supportive manner. 'They're too far from the sea.'

'Give it a try. They're delicious.' Jagu pushes the platter towards Clothilde.

'I don't think I can. I know I've grown up on a farm, and I've even had to kill a rabbit or two, but I've never had to swallow anything that was still moving.' Clothilde wrinkles up her face.

'The trick is to make the whole thing one movement,' Simone says encouragingly. 'Don't leave it sitting in your mouth. Swallow as it enters.'

'Well in that case what's the point?' Clothilde shakes her head.

'The taste!' Jagu insists. 'There's nothing like it!'

'You would say that you sell them for a living.' Neven nudges his brother-in-law good-humouredly.

'Don't feel pressured tonight,' Renée reassures Clothilde as she passes the platter to the others. 'There will be plenty of other occasions to try them.'

Isla - 2018

'Your mother was mortified at the idea of eating live shellfish,' Simone recalls, 'so she skipped the oysters. She looked a little green at the large bowl of Moule Mariniere that followed, but once we reassured her that this dish had been cooked. She plucked up enough courage to taste them.' Simone shakes her head gently. 'I don't think she had ever eaten shellfish in her life and, one variety or another appeared in four out of the six courses we had that night.'

'Poor Mam, I can just imagine it. With the party in her honour, I'm sure she wouldn't have wanted to offend you all. But faced with all those unusual foods, I can see why she wouldn't want to eat them either.'

Neither of the others speak, so I continue.

'I had my own similar moment when I was living with a host family in Germany. I was working in industry for a year, during my degree, and staying with this lovely family, but one night they made me Labskaus, which is a sloppy puree of corned beef, onions, and root vegetables, with a fried egg on top. So far so good you might say, but it is served with herring and pickles. I just didn't know what to do.'

I'm not sure why I've embarked on this story. Perhaps it's because with Simone and Odile sharing their memories of Mam, I'm finding it hard to contribute to the conversation, and I actually have the French vocabulary to tell this story.

Anyway, whatever my motivations, the story is having an impact. They both seem shocked at the idea of all these flavours mixed up together.

'Foods considered to be delicacies are so region specific, aren't they? In these days of refrigerated transport, it's easy to forget how locally sourced people's diets were sixty or seventy years ago.'

'And of course, people who were teenagers during the late forties and early fifties were often trying new foods for the first time.' Simone adds, sympathetically.

Twenty-three

Isla - 2018

Back at the hotel I reflect on my first encounter with my relatives. It's clear that there is an underlying level of reserve within the individuals on this side of my family that I'm glad to say, thanks to my father's influence, wasn't dominant in the household I grew up in.

Mam undoubtedly had this side to her nature, but her childhood at the heart of Lorna's family must have given her an understanding of the importance of close bonds. She certainly formed one with Da and did her best with me.

If I'm honest, emotional reserve is a trait that I also carry, and probably contributed to my difficulties with Mam, as much as any lack of warmth from her direction.

Simone's manner is just as I'd imagined from reading her letter. It's clear that she loved my mother very much. She has a stronger sense of humour than her daughter, and I can see how much her physical limitations frustrate her now. She must have been a very vital person in her youth. I can imagine her and Mam having a lot of fun together out at the farm.

Clothilde - 1951

This is unquestionably the best present ever! Her own bicycle. The family has clubbed together to buy it. The basket on the front is nice and big, and they've invested in a set of panniers for her as well.

Their generosity is not without ulterior motives, as she will be able to run errands for them all, but for Clothilde, it will provide the complete freedom that she has longed for since she arrived.

Although she's been going up to see Simone and Neven at the farm on a regular basis, it's only been worth going if she has a free day, because the walk takes three-quarters of an hour each way. Now with a bike, she will be there in ten minutes!

The thought of being able to pop up to see Simone after school fills Clothilde with joy. The evenings have been long and lonely since she arrived. None of her classmates have wanted to include her in their social lives.

Clothilde has tried to be friendly, and a few of the girls will say hello in the corridor, but in the last few months she's overheard conversations about several outings that she has not been invited to.

Most of the boys from the local area that she would like to get to know have already left school, and Renée and Jagu have been too protective to allow her much unsupervised time.

As she pedals along Rue des Quatre Vents, Clothilde is the happiest she has been in months. She's going to be able to explore. Although the peninsula is not that big, she's only been to more distant places in the company of a relative.

Renée and Jagu regularly ask her to keep an eye on Bernard. They don't seem to understand how limiting this is. For whilst Bernard has their permission to play out in the streets with his friends, she herself must remain at home, so that he can find her.

The route she is cycling today is the most direct route to the farm, and also the most sheltered. On sunny days it is going to be glorious to cycle along the coast road with the Atlantic breeze blowing in her hair.

Suddenly, she's on the ground, amidst a cacophony of loud squawking and flapping wings. She has cycled straight into a flock of geese milling across the road.

She picks up her brand-new bike and checks it for dents, whilst several of the geese peck at her legs. She kicks out to fend them off, and then, with nothing but her pride damaged, pedals on towards Kervihan, trying to keep at least part of her mind on the road in front of her.

Isla - 2018

It was a shame that Philippe couldn't make it tonight, but it did give me a chance to start building a relationship with Simone and Odile. I know from experience that when groups are too big you don't really talk about anything other than everyday niceties and chit-chat.

From Simone's accounts, I'm beginning to build a picture of my mother as a complex young woman. On the one hand she was determined, strong and independent, with a wicked sense of humour. On the other, she fought high levels of anxiety. Her daily life had also emphasised duty. At first on a desperately understaffed farm during the war years, and later under the firm rules in her aunt Renée's household. Sadly, these last two factors seem to have gradually suppressed her sparkling sense of humour, for by the time she became a parent, there had been little sign of it.

It's clear that with only an eight-year age gap between them, Simone's relationship with Mam became more like that of an elder sister than of an aunt. It has also been a surprise, and a delight that, although Odile had not even reached her tenth birthday when Mam left, the handful of memories she has of her are strong and clear.

There was obviously a lot of love between the three of them during the 1950s. For this reason, I cannot fathom why Mam would cut herself off from her family so completely.

I'm keen to find out more about Henri, Mam's father. Simone is going to be the only person old enough to remember her brother, and with no other source, I must write down as much as she can remember before I go home. She's remarkably spritely for ninety, but I know from the sudden shock of losing Da that life can be snatched in an instant, and I can't rely on a return visit.

It feels good to wake without the ringing of an alarm clock. I pick up my mobile from the bedside table. 9am! I'm in danger of losing the morning if I lie here much longer. I dial Simone's number. A man answers.

'Oh! Good morning. Is that Philippe?'

'Yes.' A resonant baritone voice, replies.

'This is your cousin Isla.'

I wonder what he feels about having a long-lost cousin turn up.

'Oh, how lovely to speak to you.'

Well, that's all right then. No need for me to be anxious.

'Isla, I'm going to be late for work, so I can't talk now, but are you free on Saturday to have lunch in Port Maria?'

'That would be great. I look forward to meeting you. Before you hang up, is Simone there?'

'I'll pass you over.'

'Hi Simone, sorry to call so early, but I was wondering if you would like to go on a drive with me today. I would like to talk some more, and I was hoping you could show me some of the places where Mam liked to spend time. There will be no need to step out of the car unless you would like to.'

I hold my breathe in hope. I don't know if Simone goes out very much. Perhaps this is a reckless suggestion. But I don't really see what harm sitting in a car can do.

'There's nothing I would like more.'

Simone is brisk and to the point.

'See you in an hour.'

I pull up outside Simone's house and she is already on the roadside, sitting on a walker that doubles as a seat.

'Can you fit this in the back? It will mean I can explore a little with you.'

'Of course,' I say opening the boot.

Our first stop is the car park at Plage du Conguel.

'I would often find your mother here if she was upset.' Simone tells me as we step out of the car. 'I think, in her mind, she was trying to escape the new situation she found herself in by physically taking herself as far away from everyone as she could. The tracks here lead down to the very tip of the peninsula.

As we walk slowly together along the tarmac, I can see the vast expanse of Quiberon Bay stretching off to the left, and if I glance over my right shoulder, I can just see the buildings of Port Maria in the distance.

I can see why Mam chose here to get away from it all.

Clothilde - 1956

It's Sunday, and Simone and Neven are attending a celebration for a friend in Kervihan, so they've agreed to lend Clothilde the cart. It was a little difficult helping James up into the back, but he is now happily watching the scenery disappearing away from him, as she guides the horse along the shore road.

When they reach the turn that leads out to the point, Clothilde pulls the cart in under the shade of the trees and hitches the horse to a branch. James has already wiggled himself to the edge of the cart and is lowering himself gently to the ground.

The doctor has conceded that his collarbone and shoulder are now healed enough for him to use crutches over short distances, and he obviously can't wait to get down to the water's edge.

Clothilde hurries to catch up with him as he swings himself along and leads the way down the small incline onto the Plage du Conguel. What neither of them have considered is the way that the crutches focus James's weight. As he swings out for the first time over the soft sand, the crutches disappear into the ground beneath him, throwing him off balance and onto Clothilde. The pair of them crash in a tangled heap to the ground.

'Oh, my goodness,' Clothilde shrieks, as she raises herself on her arms to look at him. 'Are you all right? Has it broken again?'

James is laughing hysterically, with his bad leg outstretched across Clothilde's thigh. His newly healed arm is buried deep in a sand dune under her shoulder, and the two offending crutches are planted firmly in the sand behind them, like gateposts.

'I'm fine. I'm fine!' he reassures her, before recovering himself enough, to appreciate the rather compromising position in which they are lying. Glancing around to see if the other people on the beach are looking, he quickly rolls his hips so that his leg swings down onto the sand beside her, and she is free to slide away from him.

He extracts his arm from the deep soft sand and looks up at Clothilde. She is chuckling quietly, as she tugs at one of the crutches.

'How much do you weigh?! These are completely stuck.'

James rolls onto his stomach. He wriggles like a snake with his left hand outstretched, until he can reach the other crutch. Grasping the part nearest the ground, he uses his free hand to excavate the sand around the wood.

Clothilde adopts the same technique, and within minutes both crutches are free and lying across James' lap, as he sits in the sand.

'What are we going to do?' she asks. 'I'm not strong enough to carry you.'

'It may not be very dignified, but I'll slide myself up the slope on my bottom. Once we're nearer the top, the ground will be firm enough to bear my weight without the crutches sinking in. I'll need a bit of help, but it should be ok because I'll have the slope in my favour.'

Clothilde jumps up, watching him anxiously, waiting for the moment that she's needed. It's obvious from the look on his face that James would rather not have the scrutiny.

From the top of the slope, he gives a nod to show that he's ready, and she climbs up herself, placing her feet firmly, one at the base of each crutch.

In one quick movement James pulls himself to standing. They are momentarily nose-to-nose, and then, as James completes the action, Clothilde's face becomes buried in his chest.

Feeling the unwelcome pull of gravity Clothilde throws her weight forward up the slope, and flings her arms around James, encircling the crutches in the process just managing to prevent them both toppling back down to the beach.

She ought to let go at once. She knows that she should, but he smells so wonderful, and she can hear his heart beating fast in his chest, because her ear is pressed against his shirt.

She pulls back, turning her head to look at him, but still doesn't let go. She tells herself that she wants to be sure that he has found his balance, but he's looking down at her, with an intensity, and a longing, which matches the way that she feels inside.

She looks frankly back at him for a moment, and then smiles as she steps away.

'I think you'll have to wait a bit longer to commune with the water. But we can take the footpath out to the point. It will be firm enough, and there are lots of boulders we can sit on if you want a rest. It will be quiet, not many people bother to walk that far at this time of day. I go there a lot if I want to be alone.'

James' eyes open wide as he hurries after her on his crutches.

Isla - 2018

The next place on Simone's tour is Plage du Drehen. This time we park where we can see the beach below us.

The tide is out and there are children building sandcastles and exploring the newly filled rock pools. A small group of men in waders are scrabbling around at the water's edge. I'm not sure if they're hunting for crabs, or shellfish, but there is a purpose about their actions that suggests locals, rather than holidaymakers.

Simone is tired, so we decide to stay in the car and talk.

Simone - 1955

As in past summers, Simone is watching Clothilde play with Odile on the beach, whilst she herself takes a well-earned rest. She's lying on a towel with a large straw hat over her face, doing her best to ignore the shouts of joy, and fake pleas from her four-year-old daughter, as she asks to be rescued. Simone smiles. Clothilde has buried Odile up to her neck in the sand and is building a giant fortress all around her.

The degree to which Clothilde missed out on a childhood has become increasingly clear. Odile's carefree abandon is obviously strange to her cousin. It's wonderful to watch this gangly teenage woman learning to let go and be spontaneous.

Renée and Jagu did a wonderful job of ensuring that Clothilde paid attention to her studies, despite her insistence at the time, that all she wanted to do was work on the farm. Now that she's left school, Renée has been making sure that she knows how to run a household for when she marries. However, Simone is unsure whether marriage will be in Clothilde's future.

For Clothilde to receive a proposal of marriage, she would first need to be spending time with young men of her own age, and as far as Simone is aware, this is not happening.

She must ask Neven if he can think of any young men who might suit her rather prickly niece. Compared to the other girls in the area Clothilde is wary and suspicious of people's motives. This is not altogether surprising, given the hard time she received about the way that she spoke when she first moved here. The girls in her class were merciless.

There had been an awful day when Simone had seen the bullying first hand. It was a few months after Clothilde first arrived. They were due to go to the seed merchants together and, as Simone was taking the cart, she had pulled up a short way from the school in a nearby square.

From her vantage point in the driver's seat, she could see Clothilde approaching from a long way down the road.

A group of girls were following behind her, throwing screwed up paper at her back. One then ran past, and deliberately knocked into her as she went, whilst another yanked Clothilde's bag from her shoulder, so that she was pulled off balance.

The whole episode was over before they reached the square, and Clothilde didn't say a thing to her aunt as she climbed up into the cart beside her.

Later, back at the farm, Simone had asked her how she was managing at school, but Clothilde pretended that everything was ok.

Simone didn't want to push too hard if Clothilde didn't want to talk about it, as they still didn't know each other very well. So, instead, she had asked Renée to be alert for the girls at school teasing Clothilde. However, her sister, clearly distracted, just mumbled something about teenage girls and sorting out the leader of the pack.

Six weeks later, Clothilde had arrived on Simone's doorstep, exhausted and distressed, with a large rip in her school shirt, having run all the way from the school to the farm. After mopping up her tears, Simone had finally persuaded her to talk.

Over a cup of coffee, Clothilde finally explained that when she first started at the school, not only had all the students had difficulty understanding her thick Auvergne accent, but most of the staff had as well. She was constantly asked to repeat herself by the teachers, and the students took up the cry wherever she went.

This had escalated to physical bullying by the third day, and she had endured it silently ever since.

Simone had been shocked that Clothilde had suffered so much before speaking up, and the very next day she and Renée had gone together to speak to the headmistress. The situation had become bearable for Clothilde from then onwards, but the damage had been done to relationships with the young people of her own age in the region.

Isla - 2018

Simone is enjoying the support of the car's headrest as she soaks in the view.

'Your mother and I used to bring Odile here to play. It was the closest beach, with calm water and decent sand. They were so sweet together. Clothilde would take Odile off looking for shrimp in the rock pools and collecting shells.'

I can just imagine the two of them playing happily down on the sand.

'However, when your mother first arrived, and Odile was a tiny baby, she had never seen the sea before, and didn't really know how to behave. She found the vast expanse of the ocean scary, and despite all my efforts, I could never persuade her to put her face in the water and swim. She would happily wade up to her waist to play with a ball, or bounce Odile in the shallows, but I could never get her to swim.'

'That's odd. Mam was quite a strong swimmer.'

'Oh, that was down to your father.'

James - 1956

Finally, James' leg is healing. He has graduated from crutches to a stick, and whilst he's allowed to put weight on his bad leg for short periods of walking, he has been told that the best rehabilitation would be swimming. So today for the first time, they are going to give it a go.

The tide is out, and James and Clothilde are resting on a large rock on Plage du Drehen. Walking through the soft sand has been tiring for James, but really, it's just an excuse to lie on the warm rock in the afternoon sun, with their heads close together, and their fingertips touching.

It's too public here to risk more, but since their first kiss at Pointe du Conguel a few weeks ago, it has been unbearable to be close, and yet unable to hold each other.

Clothilde has talked excitedly about their plan to swim, and yet now she seems anxious. Perhaps she's shy that he will be seeing her in her bathing suit. Personally, he can't wait for the moment to arrive.

The yearning to reach for her is overwhelming and, before it transfers itself to a more obvious physical display of lust, he jumps up, declaring that it is time for the serious work of the afternoon, his rehabilitation.

James has planned ahead and pulls off his shirt and trousers to reveal a pair of blue knitted swimming trunks with a white belt. He's quite pleased with them, having searched all the shops for some that will hold their shape, and not embarrass him like the ones he has at home, knitted by his mother.

Clothilde is looking uncertain as she pulls a towel from her bag, and he realises that she might not have her suit on underneath her dress.

'Why don't I make my way down to the water? It will take me a while even with my stick, and you can catch me up.'

James is normally a confident swimmer. He loves the water and can't wait to relax against its supportive fluid form. However, he's a little uncertain whether his shoulder and his leg will cooperate with his plans.

Luckily the water here is calm, and with a little help from Clothilde, he is confident that he can manage without his stick. He casts it aside and takes a further two steps so that the water is lapping at his ankles.

It's cool, but nothing like the biting temperatures he's used to in Scotland. Suddenly, he feels a warm hand around his waist, and another on his arm, as Clothilde steps into the water alongside him.

'Can I help you go deeper?' she asks.

James swallows. All he can do is nod and move forward, leaning unnecessarily on the beautiful girl in the red bathing suit, who is looking up at him intensely from under his shoulder.

They make their way out until they are waist deep, at which point Clothilde stops. James doesn't want to let go of her, but if they remain here, he will have to.

What he really wants is for them to walk on out until they are up to their necks in the water, where no one on shore will know what they are doing with their hands. He tries to encourage her to walk on with him, but for some reason she won't.

Eager not to offend her, he quickly steps from her grasp and is surprised when she looks disappointed.

'Do you want to try a few strokes?' Clothilde asks hesitantly. 'Perhaps you could go along shore rather than out to sea.'

'Where's the fun in that?' James says, quickly launching himself into deeper water, hoping that she will follow. However, she stays exactly where she is.

'What's the matter?' he shouts swimming back towards her.

'I know I'm supposed to be here for your safety,' she says 'but you're doing fine. I'll just watch from here.'

'What're you talking about? You're right. I'm more than fine. This feels great. I've not had this much freedom of movement in weeks.'

James duck dives down under the water, and holding his breath, swims back towards the shore until he can see her feet. Then he pops up right under her nose.

Startled, she falls over backwards and swallows a large mouthful of water. She regains her balance, coughing and spluttering, and very distressed.

'Don't do that!' Clothilde shouts. Striking out at him.

James steps back giving her an assessing look.

'You can't swim, can you?'

Clothilde's arms slump to her sides, and with her eyes firmly fixed on the sea in front of her, she shakes her head.

'Then we are going to have a lot of fun whilst I teach you.' James says as he steps forward and places his hands on her shoulders.

Twenty-four

Isla - 2018

I look across at Simone, who has fallen silent. She has a faraway look in her eyes, and then, all of a sudden, she becomes very animated.

'Isla, if you have time, I hope you might drive me to Carnac. It will only take forty minutes if we're lucky with the traffic.'

'Of course, with pleasure. I've nothing else to do whilst I'm here, other than spend time getting to know you. What would you like to do once we get there?'

'I want to show you where your grandfather was born. The Marec side of our family are originally from Carnac, but our parents moved here at the end of the First World War. Mother wanted to be closer to her parents, before Renée was born.'

I can't believe that once again, I've forgotten this other important strand of my search. Simone holds the key to my mother's early life, but she is also the only person still alive who knows anything about my grandfather. I can't wait to find out more.

'How old were you when Henri was killed?' I ask tentatively.

'I was twelve. He was my big brother and I idolised him. I was devastated when he died. But if I'm honest I'd been used to daily life without him. He left home when I was a toddler, and although he came back to visit, we never had extended time together. However, I do have plenty of memories of him sitting around our dinner table, telling us stories of his life in Paris.'

'How long was he there before war broke out?'

'Oh, Henri had wanted to work the railways for as long as anyone can remember, so in 1931 he made the move to Paris. I was only three.'

I can't help noticing the tone of regret in Simone's voice.

'He had been working for the railway locally before that, so it didn't take him long to reach a position of trust in the capital.'

'Were other members of the family on the railways?'

'No, not at all. Our maternal grandfather was a fisherman. He spent a long time trying to persuade Henri to follow in his footsteps. He had won the battle with our father, but Henri wasn't interested.

He got seasick out on the water and had always had a fascination for trains. He was obsessed with the connectedness of the railways, and how much of the world could be seen by travelling on the tracks.

When he moved to Paris he took a room in a boarding house near Gare du Nord, which proved very lucky for him, as that was where he met your grandmother.'

As I hear Simone talk of Henri's decisions, I feel the return of a level of peace within myself that has been absent for many months. My decision to move away to Germany and develop an independent life may not be so common in the wider world, but it obviously runs strong in the genes from my mother's side of the family.

Henri and Camille both moved to Paris against the advice and guidance of their families, and Mam herself moved to Scotland for a fresh start against the wishes of her Breton relatives.

My move to Germany was just the most recent in a long line of such decisions.

Henri - 1933

Henri is in a hurry. Gaston is waiting for him back at the station. He and his wife are on their way to a club. She's bringing her sister, and they want him to make up a four. He only popped back to change.

In his hurry to lock the door he fumbles his key, and it falls to the floor. As he bends down, through the banisters, he catches sight of a beautiful head of dark, wavy hair coming up the communal staircase towards him. The body beneath is moving with a captivating, undulating bounce.

He runs his hands through the longer, top section of his own blonde hair. It doesn't seem to matter how much pomade he uses, the front portion always seems to have a mind of its own.

Satisfied that all is in place, he smooths down his jacket, and stands ready to greet the woman as she steps forward onto the landing.

'Good evening, can I help you?' he asks as an opening line.

'Oh, good evening, no thank you, I'm fine.'

The woman continues as if to walk past him. Unwilling to let this opportunity slip away Henri continues.

'Are you looking for someone in the building? I know most of the residents.'

'Obviously, not all of us,' she answers somewhat acerbically. 'I live upstairs.'

'You do?' Henri is both shocked and delighted. 'Forgive me. Welcome! My name is Henri Marec. I'm very pleased to meet you.'

The woman looks at his outstretched hand and seems reluctant to take it, but eventually politeness forces her to grasp hold, and with a curt shake and a bob of her head, she replies.

'Camille Guery.'

'What do you do, Camille Guery, that brings you to live alone in an apartment in Paris?'

'I'm not alone,' she replies, indignant at the implication. 'I share with two of the other secretaries.'

Henri could kick himself for his crassness. He has spent too much time with only male company.

'Oh, you work with Micheline and Eloise at head office?' Hopefully showing to her that he knows her colleagues will reassure her that he is in fact, all right.

'I do. Now if you'll excuse me, I'm in rather a hurry.' And with that she is gone, around the bend and up the next flight of stairs, leaving Henri with a lasting memory of a very shapely pair of legs, disappearing from view.

Needless to say, Gaston's sister-in-law didn't stand a chance that night. It's taken him three weeks, but Henri has persuaded Camille to accept his advances, and now they spend every evening together.

Tonight, they are in the small bistro on Rue Muller.

'They're moving me tomorrow,' Henri breaks his news nonchalantly. 'I won't be on the Calais service any longer.'

'Really?' Camille appears to be feigning a similar degree of disinterest. 'Which line will you be on?'

'The route to Lile.' He watches as she gives him the smallest of nods. 'The journeys will be a lot shorter, which will allow me more time to work for them at the office.'

The corners of her mouth flick with a suppressed smile.

'Apparently, someone has told head office that I speak several languages!' He purses his lips and gives Camille a pointed stare. 'They want me to translate some of the paperwork.'

Cracking under his gaze she drops her act.

'Well, you do, don't you? You told me that you've picked up German, Swiss-German, Dutch, Flemish, English, and Italian all since you started working the trains.'

'Yes, but I don't have any official qualifications.'

'I can't see how that matters.' Camille reassures him, as she reaches across the restaurant table to seductively sip his drink.

Isla - 2018

The traffic has ground to a halt, so I take the chance to ask a further question of Simone.

'How well did you know my grandmother?'

'Camille only came to Quiberon a few times. The first was in 1934, when I was six years old. We organised a big family party to celebrate their engagement. Camille was so beautiful. I thought my brother was marrying a princess. I know everyone always says that brides-to-be are beautiful, but your grandmother really was stunning.'

I wonder where that stunning Guery beauty came from. I think it must have been Joseph's family, because according to Lorna, Chloe thought herself ugly and from the photographs that I've seen at Odile's house, and Philippe's, both my mother and I take after the Marec side of the family, in terms of appearance.

Camille - 1934

Camille is nervous as she steps through the doorway into the crowded hall. Although she and Henri have been together for eighteen months, this is the first opportunity that she's had to meet his family. There are so many of them.

Clusters of people of all ages are deep in conversation, drinks in hand. Two rather harassed looking teenagers, each with a babe in arms, are supervising a group of young children sitting around a table at the far end of the room.

As the only child of only children, the thought of so much extended family is quite overwhelming. That they all live so close together, is suffocating. She totally understands why Henri headed for Paris as soon as he could.

Henri - 1934

Henri looks around at the hall. It has been specially decorated in their honour by his sisters. They've done him proud. It looks beautiful. His arm tightens around Camille's waist, and he guides her forward into the crowd, beaming with pride. No one can question his decision to leave for the capital, now. There's not a woman in the room who can match his fiancée in appearance.

Camille is wearing a brand-new dress, from a renowned boutique in Paris, she has saved up all her wages for the last six months to afford it, and with her natural poise and grace she is a magnet to his relatives.

However, unfortunately, as the night goes on, it seems that Camille's appearance and demeanour are not bringing the uniform warm responses that he had hoped for. The men are all smitten. Many have come up to shake his hand, and slap him on the back at his luck, but he can see the women looking at her out of the corner of their eyes as she moves around the room. It is not admiration that he sees on their faces.

Most of the women here are wives and mothers. They make their own clothes and work hard looking after their families. None of them would spend the time that Camille does on their appearance, or on reading books to develop their minds. They know nothing of the hours of pleasure he has with Camille, back home in Paris, discussing books.

Isla - 2018

Simone makes a slight sucking noise through her teeth.

'I believe that engagement party was responsible for opening my sister Renée's eyes to the woman that she wanted to become.' Simone says biting her lower lip in thought.

"I don't understand.'

'We were all pretty provincial here in Quiberon, until your grandmother came to visit. Renée was fourteen years old and very impressionable. Camille arrived with great taste in clothes, a passion for literature and learning, and a natural preference for sophistication and elegance in her surroundings.'

'So, the house that you now live in with Philippe?'

'All those fine furnishings, and shelves full of books, were acquired by my sister once she got married. She was determined to reinvent herself in Camille's image. Our family naturally had much more humble tastes, and I have to admit that I always felt much more relaxed up at the farm.'

'But didn't Camille grow up on a farm too?'

I know that my grandmother had very humble origins in Barantan, however, Simone's description does fit with something that Lorna said, about how she dressed.

'There was just something burning inside Camille, which sought out adventure, and status, and acclaim, and it had nothing to do with her upbringing.'

My grandmother sounds quite a force of nature. I wish I could have known her. The feisty little eight-year-old me would have loved to meet her, desperate as she was to find her place in the wider world. I'm certain that Camille would also have understood the business me, who wore designer outfits, and chose to live in a luxury apartment.

However, Simone's next words suggest that she doesn't view these characteristics in quite the same positive light that I do.

'Whilst she was here, Camille talked very scathingly about the way that her parents tried to contain her in their small village. Apparently, they had plans for her to marry the son of a local farmer. Her father had begun talking to the celebrant and deciding without her, so one night, she packed her bags, and the next morning she hitched a lift to town and followed the railway to Paris.'

'You mean she ran away from home?'

This would have made their daughter's wartime disappearance a repeat experience for Joseph and Chloe. It must have been agony. I can't believe Lorna didn't tell me this part of the story. Perhaps she didn't know.

After all, it happened before she was born, and possibly before Rory and Dominique had moved to the area.

I can't make up my mind how I feel about my grandmother. Simone certainly thinks she was egotistical and possibly even narcissistic, and yet, I have to admire her feminist drive. A quality that would not have been common in women of her era.

She appears to have had an enthusiastic determination to live a life, carved out by her own actions, as she followed her dreams.

Lorna had nothing bad to say about her. But I guess she was only a child when Camille returned to Barantan. In my experience, childhood impressions of other people are rarely kept unless they are strongly positive, or strongly negative. Also, Lorna would have had little contact with Camille before her disappearance, as she was based in Vichy most of that time.

There are undeniable parallels between Camille's life choices and my own. I wonder if other people judge my decision to leave West Kilbride in a similar way.

Twenty-five

Isla - 2018

Philippe and I are sitting in the shade of a large umbrella, outside a seafood restaurant in Port Maria, supposedly so that I can look out across the harbour. But I can't take my eyes off my cousin's hands.

They are Mam's hands! Larger of course, as they are attached to a broad-shouldered man in his mid-fifties, but with the same over-all proportions, shape of nails, and curve in the little fingers.

He also gesticulates with them as he speaks, in the same way that she did. He lifts one hand now to sweep an errant lock of light brown hair from his eyes, and it makes me want to cry at the similarities between him and Mam. For his hair, like Mam's and mine, was obviously blonde. I cheat and continue to dye mine, but over time we have all darkened from the white blonde of our youth. It would have been wonderful if Philippe and Mam could have met. It's such a shame!

With every day that passes, I find it harder and harder to understand why Mam cut herself, and by extension me, from our family. They are such nice people. Our lives could have been so different with French relatives to visit.

With a wider sense of family, perhaps I would have felt a little less alone and on the outside of my parents' intense relationship, although if I'm honest, my preference for solitude is more likely inherited from my father, than generated by exclusion.

During outings in my childhood, Da would usually head to the far end of the beach for time alone, whilst Mam and I set up camp and unpacked the picnic. When the time was right, I would be sent to collect him.

These mental images of Da as a solitary figure are at least as strong as the delightful ones I have of the two of us building sandcastles, and rock-pooling together.

Philippe has started speaking. I must pay attention.

'So, I gather that your mother came to live here with my father and my grandparents in the early 1950s. It's ridiculous. I didn't know she even existed. They never talked about her.'

This news makes me feel cold. Ok, Mam chose to leave and break contact, but for the family to also pretend that she had never existed seems harsh and rejecting. Especially as they were all living together with an obvious space where she used to be.

'Really?' I ask. 'Not ever?'

'Not that I remember, but then she had been gone more than ten years by the time I was old enough to remember conversations amongst the adults in my life. Plus, my father was never one to talk about his feelings. Not even when my mother died. I was twelve and my father dealt with that in a similar way, as if she had never existed. He just drew a line and moved on.'

This approach to emotional distress seems to be a family trait! Perhaps it's the key to how this whole estrangement came about. If every family member closed down, and kept their feelings to themselves after the separation, it is easy to see how Mam's memory got lost to the next generation, and how I in turn, failed to hear about them.

But Simone hadn't accepted Mam's absence as a painful thing to lock away, she had written to her. Surely, she would have spoken to the others about Mam? But then again, events seem to have a terrible way of repeating themselves in this family, and maybe circumstances overtook everyone.

It's awful that Philippe also lost his mother so young, and that Bernard refused to talk about her is unforgivable.

'I'm so sorry Philippe, I can't believe that your father did that. As a teenager, did you have anyone to talk to? Simone and Odile both seem a little more family-orientated?'

I am surprised by his reply.

'Odile had moved away by that time, and Neven was sick, so Simone was running the farm pretty much single-handed. She was always kind, and supportive, if we went there, but she didn't have time to visit us. My sister and I pretty much stuck together. We were sixteen months apart, but although I was older, she was female and more emotionally mature. In many ways, we behaved more like twins. Where one went, the other went too.'

'Your sister?' This is a shock to me. 'Is she still alive?'

'Of course! Did Odile not mention her?'

Philippe seems quite upset that I don't know about his sister.

'I suppose there has been so much to share that we haven't got to her yet.'

Even to me this doesn't sound good. *Out of sight out of mind* seems to be a thing in this family!

'That sounds bad. I just mean that I met Odile when I was looking for Simone in Kervihan. She then told me about you, because Simone was living with you, and I learnt about Bernard and your grandparents all living in that house, but I haven't got on to wider family yet.'

He seems to be calming down, so I forge on.

'What's her name? Does she live locally? I'd love to meet her.'

'I invited her today, but they had a university event in Brest that they had to go to.'

'They?'

'My sister, Fabienne, is married to Erwan, who's a lecturer at the Centre for Breton and Celtic Research up in Brest. They've got two daughters. Rozenn is also in Brest. She's following in her father's footsteps studying something they call *Languages, Literature & Foreign & Regional Civilizations*, it's a ridiculous mouthful. Their other daughter Nolwenn is unfortunately studying abroad at the moment, so you won't be able to meet her.'

So many names. So many facts, with nothing to pin them to. Is this how Mam felt? Was her brain filled with unconnected pieces of information all searching for a home where they would make sense?

I've already forgotten what his sister and her husband are called. In fact, the only one I can remember is Nolwenn, and she's the one who's not here! Where is that family tree when I need it?

'I'd love for you to meet them.' Philippe continues. 'Can you come to the house tomorrow evening for dinner? They'll be back by then. I promise not to cook. I'll buy some ready prepared food from the delicatessen.'

'That would be wonderful.'

I take out a tissue and wipe at the corners of my eyes before the tears can fall. A warm feeling of hope and belonging is flooding through my body.

Family.

It's a word I thought I'd lost, and now it seems to just keep on growing.

Isla - 2018

It's Sunday night, and I arrived a little early for dinner, intending to help prepare the meal. Instead, Philippe had another idea. We are currently sitting on the floor in his attic, with a small inlaid and lacquered box between us.

'My grandmother kept some of the letters that were special to her in this,' Philippe says, as he opens the box. 'I know they are not all from my grandfather. There are a couple written on violet notepaper, which I thought might have been from a woman. Look, here they are.'

I reach forward and take a fragile looking letter from his outstretched hand. I unfold it, and there at the bottom is the signature - Camille.

'Can we take it downstairs and read it? I might need Odile's help with the translation.'

'Of course. Let's take this one as well. It's on the same paper.'

I take a seat on the sofa next to Odile. Simone is in her usual chair, and Philippe is arranging drinks-glasses and nibbles over in the corner.

'It's a letter to Renée, from Paris. I think it was sent not long after the engagement party that you told me about, Simone.'

Camille - 1934

Camille is lying on the sofa in her apartment. Her head resting in Henri's lap.

'You promised me a new poet today, what have you got?' she asks reaching up and twisting an errant lock of his honey-blond hair in her fingers.

'It's a treat, but you're going to have to work hard for it. These poems are in German.'

Camille pulls a face.

'But you'll translate them for me?'

'*With* you.' Henri corrects. 'This is a chance for us to continue your German lessons. *You* are going to look at the text, as *I* hold it here in front of us. Listen to the pronunciation as I read the words aloud. Then afterwards, I will translate each poem, so that you can understand how marvellous it is.'

'So, who is this great master?' she teases. Nudging him gently with her elbow.

'The poems are called Neue Gedichte, and they are by Rainer Maria Rilke. Although they're written in German, he wrote them whilst living here in Paris. The second volume is dedicated to Rodin. He greatly influenced Rilke. We should try and see some of his sculpture if we can. It will help us understand the poems.'

Camille wriggles with excitement.

'I can't wait to write to Renée. She's always desperate to know how we've spent the evening. She will be so envious. Poor thing, she can't wait to be old enough to join us here in Paris. We can make that happen for her, can't we Henri?'

Henri is not so keen on the idea of having his little sister in Paris. He has said, more than once, that he could do without the responsibility.

'Luckily, we don't have to make that decision just yet. She's only fourteen.'

'But she's suffocating out there on that peninsula. Renée has a mind, and she wants to use it.'

'Well, let's concentrate for now on your mind, and putting that to good use.' Henri says, as he places his long index finger under the first line of text and begins to read aloud.

Isla - 2018

The quiet that fell over the room as I started to read is broken by a sudden guffaw.

'So that's how Renée developed her obsession with foreign literature.' Simone is chuckling as she speaks. 'None of us could ever work it out. I should have known it was Camille.'

Philippe chimes in from his position by the window.

'I remember grandmother going to enormous trouble to have books sent to her from the foreign language bookshops in Paris. In the last few years, she would often ask me to place the orders for her.'

'Quite a lot of them are still here on the shelves.' Odile says, as she stands up and crosses to the bookcase.

'Look, here's a volume of Rilke poetry.' She opens it. 'Renée has written her name and the date she got it, February 1935.'

'That's so ridiculous. She didn't even speak German then. Why on earth was she spending her money on that?' Simone shakes her head, puzzled by her sister's ways.

'She just wanted to be like her brother's future wife.' Odile says with more than a shade of understanding.

'I think she was more in love with Camille than Henri was.' Simone laughs dismissively.

It's a throw away statement, but I wonder if there might actually have been a grain of truth in it. Might Renée have been in love with her brother's fiancée? A preference for women would not have been something a young teenager would have wanted to share with her provincial relatives. Whatever the truth of her feelings for Camille, Renée had definitely been envious of her lifestyle and freedom.

'So, what about the other letter, what does it say?' Simone is impatient to learn more.

'It's dated much later, July 1936.'

Camille - 1936

Camille and Henri are across the river from Chateau de la Roche-Guyon. The ruined dungeon spirals up the steep hillside, appearing to grow directly out of The River Seine. Vast and imposing from any point in the valley.

'This must be where Braque stood to paint it.' Camille says excitedly. 'Look, here's the sketch I did when we saw it at the hanging. It lines up.'

'Well, aren't you the clever one? So, now that we have satisfied your intellect, and traced one of the earliest Cubist pictures to its origins, can we go for a swim? I'm boiling, and the river looks so inviting.' Henri pleads.

'Perhaps. I can't believe this is the same river that flows past us in the centre of Paris, you'd never catch me swimming there.' Camille comments.

Henri reaches for her hand and pulls her along towards the bridge. This is the first time that they've taken advantage of the new holiday laws. He means to make the most of their time. Cycling in the forest, some visits to the local churches, and of course an abundance of candlelit dinners and steamy nights in their hotel room.

Many of his friends are saving extra money by going camping, but there is no way that Camille would ever agree to sleep in a tent. There is a literal price to be paid to have the most fabulous woman in France as his wife, and he is willing to pay it.

Isla - 2018

I look up from the letter slightly puzzled.

'Can anyone explain to me what she means by the new holiday laws?'

Simone comes to my rescue.

'In May of 1936 the Popular Front came to power in France, and one of the first things that they did was to introduce paid holidays for all employees. The lack of paid holiday was one of the main reasons we saw so little of Henri once he moved to Paris.'

'In this letter Camille refers to her husband. So, at some point, in between the two letters, they got married.'

'That was the only other time I met Camille.' Simone's voice is full of regret.

'They got married here in Quiberon.'

This is not what I had expected her to say.

'The story was that Camille's parents disapproved of Henri, so they weren't invited. However, I'm not sure that was the full story. Renée and I discussed Camille often during the war. As you can imagine, we were devastated that she hadn't brought Clothilde here to live with us as planned. Renée was so used to receiving regular letters, from the woman that she idolised, that she was lost without them.'

Once again, the bitterness creeps in, as Simone talks about the relationship between my grandmother and her sister.

'She would read, and re-read, the collection of letters that she had, taking every opportunity to speak Camille's name out loud. However, my comments always infuriated her. I thought that Camille had an image that she liked to portray, that would have been tarnished by her parents' humble farming background. Those origins didn't quite fit with the identity that she had constructed for herself.'

'But our family were no further up the social hierarchy.' Philippe interjects.

'That's true,' Simone continues, 'and it's a big part of why I came to the conclusions that I did. Camille took no trouble to hide her distain for our relatives. The difference was that we were Henri's family, and not a direct reflection on her.'

I am struck by the vehemence of Simone's answers. The two women had obviously clashed much more deeply that their brief connections might imply. I wonder if there was an element of jealousy. Perhaps Simone felt that she lost her big sister to Camille, the day that she arrived, and Renée shifted her focus to the wider world.

The doorbell rings and I'm quite glad to shift the focus of our conversation away from Camille. She seems to have been quite a controversial figure within the family.

Philippe returns from the hallway followed by a petite, dark haired woman of my own age, who must be Fabienne, and a mousey haired man of about five foot ten, with a pointed face, and wire-framed glasses, who must be her husband.

I have a sudden panic, as I can't remember his name. I know it was unusual to my ears. He is followed into the room by one of his daughters, a young woman with similar hair colouring and a tall, slim frame.

Fabienne walks straight up to me, places her arms around me in a firm hug, and says clearly into my ear, 'Welcome to the family.'

Perhaps I am growing used to these hugs, or to being part of an extended family, or maybe it's because I instantly like this woman, but whatever the reason, I am delighted by her greeting.

'Fabienne, it's so lovely to meet you.' I reply looking anxiously over her shoulder at her husband.

Philippe comes to my rescue with introductions.

'Isla, this is Erwan and Rozenn. As you know sadly Nolwenn is away studying at the moment, so we will have to find another time for you to meet her.'

We all exchange greetings, and once again I embark on the story of how I found Odile.

Isla - 2018

I'm driving into Saint Julien on my way to visit Fabienne, for a guided tour of her home village, when my mobile rings.

'Isla, I'm so sorry. I've been delayed. I'll be another half an hour. Can you begin without me?'

'Of course.' I say, although I am slightly disappointed that our time alone has been cut short. 'Phone me when you arrive, and I'll tell you where I am.'

Without my guide, I decide to start with the most obvious landmark, the beautiful little chapel that I passed a moment ago. With a bit of luck, it might be open.

Clothilde - 1951

Clothilde slowly descends the staircase, enjoying the solitude, and the way that her spirit seems to expand into the empty rooms around her. For the first time since she arrived in Brittany a couple of months ago, Renée and Jagu have agreed to leave her alone at home, whilst they take Bernard out for the day.

The whole village is quiet. It is still early for a Sunday morning, but she is restless and in need of a walk.

She heads up Rue des Quatre Vents with a view to visiting the farm. It's only when she has already walked as far as Kerné that she remembers that Neven has taken Odile and Simone to visit his great-aunt today.

Deciding to explore new territory, Clothilde turns right towards the sheltered coast, and the string of villages that she has been told are dotted all along the bay. Before long she sees a sign, Saint Julien, one and a half kilometres. That will do.

As she enters the village she can see a spire above the rooftops, and she's drawn towards the church, where a service is about to begin.

Although she has never attended church regularly, Clothilde has always found churches to be peaceful places, and with no specific plans for the day, she decides to follow the final members of the congregation into the building.

As she enters, she can feel the burning penetration, as multiple sets of eyes stare at her. She is relieved that she happens to be wearing a suitable dress and her new school shoes, rather than her dirty old boots.

Clothilde slips into a pew in the back row and bows her head in respect. As the service begins, and the locals shift their focus to the front, Clothilde glances around her.

She is surprised to discover that she is in Chapelle de Saint Julien. She learned about St Julien at school because he was from Brioude in the Auvergne! Here she is, miles from home, and the first chapel that she enters is dedicated to a saint from the Auvergne.

The tears start to fall, and she bows her head once more. They are her first public tears, and yes, they are tears of sorrow, but also of relief. For although she is alone in this new part of the country, with these unfamiliar people, she has discovered a place that she can come to, that will always be able to connect her to everything that she has lost.

Clothilde had been unaware that a part of her wanted this connection. She had been trying so hard to distance herself from everything and everyone back home. Even now, she is unsure of the wisdom of letting the memories back in.

The ice is manageable, in its cold predictability. It allows her to function, on a daily basis, and to put up a front that others see as a normal person.

She knows that to come here regularly will be playing with fire. The heat from which is likely to melt the ice. But with the floodgates open, will the rivers of emotion be navigable?

Isla - 2018

I'm still in the Chapel when Fabienne joins me.

'It's easy to imagine Mam sitting here. These wooden pews, the peeling paint on the walls, even this rather odd collection of free-standing furniture. It all looks as if it's been here for decades.' I comment as I sweep my arm across in front of me.

'They have.' Fabienne acknowledges. 'There was a large fundraising effort by the locals in the 1920s to restore the chapel, but the money for its upkeep has been harder to find in recent years.'

'Do you know anything about the wooden sculpture over there?' I ask. 'It's quite scary.'

'Only that it's a sculpture of Saint Anne. I agree. It's enough to give a child nightmares. In fact, shall we head on out? It makes me feel creepy.'

I rise to follow her, and as we enter the square she continues.

'It's quite likely that Clothilde would have taken part in the big processions associated with St Julien. The feast of St Julien occurs on the Sunday closest to the 28th of August, with people dressed in traditional costume parading through the streets.'

Before I can ask whether it still takes place here, I find myself leaping out of the way of an oncoming car.

Clothilde - 1953

It has taken Clothilde a while to persuade her guardians that she can take part in the procession. But having proven to Renée that she was willing to stay up late into the night to make her own costume, and to put in several hours up at the church helping in other ways, her aunt has finally agreed.

The two halves of her heritage have aligned in this parade. She feels entitled to wear the Breton outfit of her father's ancestors, and she is commemorating the saint who spent most of his life in the region where her mother was born - and probably died.

With every step that she takes carrying her heavy banner, she feels a sense of belonging, and a growing sense of who she is. At seventeen she is a woman, and yet they all still treat her as a child. The elaborate negotiations she had to go through to take part in this parade are just one example.

She's considered leaving Renée and Jagu's house more than once, but where would she go? She has no money, and few skills. She understands farming, but these days there are plenty of strong men looking for work, and the bigger farms have got tractors and other forms of motorised equipment that mean that skill with a scythe is no longer an asset.

Life on the peninsula is essentially island life. People stay close to home, shop locally, and build their hopes and dreams locally. No one passes through. They come here deliberately, or not at all. She can count on one hand the number of times she has travelled beyond the isthmus since her arrival.

With no hope of a life on Simone and Neven's farm, her future is unlikely to be in the area, unless she marries and starts a family, and although she would like someone to love and care for, she can't imagine trusting someone else that deeply.

She's going to have to come up with a plan. But right now, she has absolutely no idea how to find a way to support herself and start a move to a new area.

Isla - 2018

During the last few days, Fabienne and I have walked most of the southern coastal paths around the peninsula. So today, we are meeting further north, at Plage de Kerbourgnec in St Pierre Quiberon.

The sun is strong, the tide is high, and the beach is crowded with tourists when we arrive. So, we retreat to a local bar for a cool drink in the hope that, as the tide goes out, there will be space for walking along the shore.

'It's a great spot for swimming,' Fabienne enthuses. 'The sea here is shallow, and there are lifeguards, and a kids club, further along the beach. Children love it. Both my girls learnt to swim here, and as you can see, it's still my own favourite for a quick dip. I hope you remembered your swimsuit.'

Clothilde - 1956

Clothilde is lying on her back, deeply aware of James' hand supporting her spine as she kicks her legs. He keeps telling her to lower her head, so that her feet can rise to the surface, but the moment her ears fill with the cold seawater, she panics.

'Let's go nearer the shore.' He suggests. 'I'll sit on the sand facing the sea and put both my arms out straight. You can then lie in the water over the top of them, so I have one arm under your shoulders, and one under your hips. You can't possibly drown in fifty centimetres of water with my arms there to catch you. You'll be practically sitting in my lap.'

Clothilde quite likes the idea of sitting in his lap, so readily agrees. Surprisingly, the approach actually seems to work, with regard to her swimming, and once she becomes accustomed to water in her ears, James persuades her to roll over and try putting her face in the water.

This, however, is one step too far, and Clothilde starts thrashing around. Within moments she is up, out of the water, and he is holding her safely in his arms. James turns around and, taking a few steps up the beach, places her gently on the firm sand at the water's edge.

Shaking and coughing she gasps for breath.

'Are you ok?' he asks.

Clothilde nods sheepishly.

'Perhaps I should stick to backstroke for a while. I think I really have got the hang of that.'

'Come on then, let's get you back in the water before you develop a phobia. We'll go waist deep this time, and you can kick all the way along the bay. I'll keep my hands under you and walk along beside you.'

Isla - 2018

I'm following Fabienne down the road, slightly regretting my decision to leave my damp swimsuit on under my sarong. She's keen to show me something but won't say what. As we approach another group of nondescript houses she calls out,

'Here we are.'

I look up at the sound of her voice. I've been walking in bare feet, with my eyes firmly fixed to the ground, watching out for sharp pebbles. I raise my gaze, to find myself staring at a substantial collection of standing stones.

The stones remind me of a herd of animals in an enclosed paddock. The land on which they stand, is completely surrounded by a well-maintained, thick green hedge, separating the stones from a ring of white, slate-roofed cottages. I am intrigued.

According to the sign, the twenty-three stones visible here, are part of a greater collection that is now covered by the sea. I can't help worrying about the impact that the salt water is having on them.

As we enter the enclosure, I come to fully appreciate the size of the stones. Many are over two metres tall. This is more like it. The ones I saw the other day out on the Côte Sauvage are puny in comparison, but perhaps they are the tail end of a trail leading towards this larger group. I must investigate that.

Clothilde - 1956

Today James has finally had permission from the doctor to use his leg for more than walking. Bernard, a tad reluctantly, has agreed to lend James his bicycle, and they are going to pack a picnic and see where the road takes them.

Clothilde is happy that this new development will give the two of them more independence. When the distances are too great for James to walk, they will no longer need to borrow the cart, or ask for a lift from Simone.

However, with every health target that James reaches, the day comes closer when he will have to leave. This is not something that Clothilde wants to think about. During the daytime she can push it to the back of her mind, but for the last few nights, she has been waking at three in the morning in an agitated state.

Unable to stay in bed, she has prowled the lower floor of her aunt's house, searching for something to take her mind off her impending loss.

This morning, it was a volume of Wordsworth's poetry that she found on her aunt's bookshelf. It included the poem *The Monument* about an ancient stone circle in the North of England, which had given her the idea to begin their ride today with a visit to see their own standing stones, up the coast at Kerbourgnec.

Not wanting to push James too hard, Clothilde sets off at a leisurely pace, but he is excited at his newly found freedom, and soon they are racing along, with the wind whipping at their hair.

She is determined not to be beaten by a man, especially one who has been bed ridden for the last six months. So, throwing all caution to the wind, she races ahead to the entrance to the standing stones.

James - 1956

James places his bicycle on the ground beside Clothilde's. He is glad to have the opportunity to rest, as the muscles of his thigh are screaming. They have not been used like this for many months.

He scans the area in search of Clothilde and is stunned to find an enormous collection of standing stones visible through a gap in the hedge. Assuming that she has gone ahead of him, he reaches for his trusty French phrase book, for he knows that it has a blank page at the front, and he wants to record these impressive stones. He tucks a pencil behind his ear as he walks into the enclosure.

Whilst this collection of stones is certainly calling out to be sketched, he has an ulterior motive for starting to draw. He can't possibly cycle any further. He needs a substantial rest if he's going to have any chance of completing their outing today. What an idiot he was to race Clothilde like that, after all these months of careful rehabilitation. If he has blown it now, he will be furious. And yet, he can't help thinking that perhaps his subconscious wants to have a setback.

These months of recuperation have been the happiest of his life, despite the disaster that instigated them. His initial anxiety, about how he would finance his recovery, was alleviated when the doctor suggested that he pay for room and board by conducting some redecoration work at the surgery.

It was an excellent plan, well within his physical capabilities. Every evening, after the patients are gone, he can now be found sanding wooden window frames, sweeping floors, or balancing up a ladder on his good leg, painting the ceilings.

Unfortunately, as his leg feels stronger, his list of jobs is getting smaller, and it is only going to be a matter of weeks, before he will need to find work away from the peninsula.

His parents have been writing, trying to persuade him to return to Scotland. They haven't understood why he failed to make the return journey as soon as he could stand. This of course is because he has said nothing about Clothilde in his letters, other than that there is a woman in the area who can translate for him.

He is unsure why he has kept his feelings for Clothilde a secret. Perhaps it is because he is still only eighteen, and his parents are likely to say that he is too young to know his own mind, or perhaps because Clothilde is his senior by two years and might not take him seriously if he suggested that their relationship could be more than just a closeness born of circumstance. Age matters less as people get older, but right now, he still has 'teen' associated with his name.

Whatever the truth, he is going to have to act soon.

'What do you think?' Clothilde steps out from behind one of the stones with her arms wide open to take in the whole group.'

'They're very impressive.'

'As is my ability to beat you on a bicycle!'

'That too!' James steps forward and pulls her towards him. The only way to take the self-satisfied grin off her face is to kiss her.

James is extremely content. For the last twenty minutes he has been sitting on the grass, his back against one of the stones, with the sun shining on his face. Clothilde has gone off in search of something for them to drink, whilst he puts pencil to paper to record their surroundings.

However, it is not long before he succumbs to his drowsiness, relishing the warmth of the sun as it penetrated his closed lids.

His peaceful reverie is shattered by Clothilde's energetic return. She is carrying a newspaper and two small bottles of lemonade.

'It's only another kilometre and then you'll see how close we are to being an island,' she is obviously raring to go. 'It does actually happen occasionally in the most powerful storms, because the water washes all the way across the road.'

Acknowledging that he has had as much rest as he's going to get, James pushes himself to standing.

It has taken him weeks to develop his understanding of the geography of this strip of land because the boat docked at Port Maria, right at the foot of the peninsula, and he was taken directly to surgery from there.

Although he has only been able to access locations a few minutes' walk from the cart, he has been surprised by the diversity of the shoreline. Every outing that he and Clothilde have taken, has revealed new gems.

In this respect, there is quite a lot of similarity between this part of Brittany and the area in Cornwall that his family fish. That too is a thin strip of land, with a rough Atlantic coast opposite a more sheltered and densely populated set of bays.

His cousins in Cornwall must by now have received notification of his accident. He really must write to them and arrange to pick up his remaining belongings. He had after all, said that he would be back to collect them a few months ago.

As they approached the isthmus, James can immediately see the differences between the landscapes of the two countries. Here in Brittany, despite the tiny distance between the two shores, the inland coast is almost like a lagoon it is so flat and calm, and yet, fifty metres to the left, the Atlantic waves are churning on the beach.

There is nowhere in Cornwall like this.

'One of these days I hope to show you my country.' James blurts out. He is taken completely by surprise, as he had promised himself, he wouldn't say anything until he was a little more certain of her feelings.

'Tell me about Britain. I only know it from poetry and folk tales.'

'Well, Cornwall is a lot like Brittany, but the villages feel more huddled together. I can't say that I have seen much else of England, but Scotland is the most beautiful place in the world. The rugged empty mountains stand up tall from the water's edge. They are wild places, where the flora and fauna live and grow with a vibrant energy that you don't find in other places.'

'I've never heard you talk like this before.' Clothilde seems surprised at his passion.

'Perhaps I've deliberately avoided thoughts of home whilst I've been in recovery. My homeland always brings it out in me.'

Clothilde - 1956

Clothilde feels a cold wave penetrate to her core. She has been kidding herself. This young Scotsman is never going to set up home in France and become a local fisherman - heading out on the trawlers from Port Maria or learning about oysters from her uncle Jago. He is going to return home to his family, and his life, in just a few weeks, and she will never see him again.

'After this afternoon I now know that standing stones are something else the two countries have in common.'

James is still speaking, unaware of the destructive force his comments are having on their budding relationship. The ice is advancing, and she is barely able to hear what he is saying.

'We have some on the Isle of Arran near where I live, we could make a trip to see them.'

Twenty-six

Isla - 2018

Today the rain is falling relentlessly. I have telephoned Simone and rescheduled our outing for tomorrow, and now I have a rare free day ahead of me.

I have updated the family tree to include Fabienne and her family, and with a bit of luck I will have received some more letter translations from Adjavella.

I check my email eagerly, and to my delight she has sent a further three translations. I have been remiss. I've failed to write to update her on my wonderful success here over the last few days. I vow to read only one letter before writing back to tell her what I have discovered since arriving in Brittany. She deserves to know. I couldn't have done any of this without her.

The letters have so much unfamiliar vocabulary, in tenses that I have yet to master, that each one would have taken me days to translate, even if I could decipher the florid handwriting.

To my surprise, I have found that speaking, in person, to everyone here has been comparatively straightforward. Perhaps it's because I often know the context for the conversation, or maybe my relatives are adjusting the vocabulary that they use when they see me struggling.

It's quite strange to use that word - relatives - as I've not really needed it before. Parents has always been sufficient in applicable situations. Now for the first time I am facing the issues of large family dynamics.

My only points of reference for these types of relationships come from works of fiction. Novels, television dramas and films all have issues that arise from misunderstandings between family members. Sibling relationships certainly seem the most fraught. They often appear clouded by history and contrasting relationships with other family members.

So, when it turns out that one of the letters Adjavella has translated for me was sent to Mam, in 1960, by Renée, I am eager to get a sense of my great-aunt through her own words, rather than through the eyes of her sister.

Dear Clothilde,

It has been a month now since you left our home, and your absence is truly felt. Neither your cousin nor your uncle is a great linguist, so I have nobody that appreciates the sound of English poetry, or is willing to sit with me, to delve into the heart of the characters from my beloved novel collection.

Those evenings spent with you were like having your mother back in my life, although of course, her intellect was far superior to either of ours.

She genuinely was the most amazing woman I have ever met. I am so sorry you never really got to know her. I did find two of her letters the other day tucked inside the cover of one of my books. I'm sorry I didn't find them sooner.

I hope you will be happy in Scotland, and perhaps now that English will be your first language, you will come across some new writers whose work we might both enjoy.

I certainly hope that when your wish for separation abates, we can resume a communication on the subject of literature.
With all good wishes,
Your aunt Renée.

Clothilde - 1952

Clothilde is sitting bolt upright on a chair to the left of the fire. In her lap she has a large dual-language dictionary, and a copy of Jane Eyre. Her aunt is settling herself in the chair opposite.

Jagu is out for the evening, which has given them the chance to settle down to Renée's favourite activity, the discussion of English literature.

'It's best if you read.' Renée admits. 'Although I find your accent difficult to understand, you're a much more fluent reader than I am, and we don't want to be stuck on the first page all night.' She leans over towards her niece. 'Pass me the dictionary. I'll look up anything that you don't know, not that that happens often. You really are very gifted at languages, unlike the men in my life.'

Clothilde passes the heavy dictionary across, looking rather apprehensively at her aunt. Whilst she enjoys having the chance to read in English, she hates having her accent corrected by someone who isn't even British.

Also, her aunt has so many expectations of how the evening will progress, that it feels very much like being in school, rather than a pleasurable way to pass the time together.

'Of course, your mother was a great linguist and an immensely cultured person altogether...'

'She was?'

Clothilde can't help but interrupt. She can feel her heart rate rising. How is it that her father's sister, a way over here in Brittany, seems to know more about Camille than either Chloe or Joseph?

'I don't really know anything about Maman, other than what my grandparents told me of her childhood in Barantan.' Clothilde confesses. 'We used to read together, and sometimes she would sing me a song as I was falling asleep. I do remember her hands. They were never muddy, even though we lived on a farm, and her nails were always long and beautifully shaped - the opposite of labourers' hands.'

'That certainly sounds like Camille. I only met your mother twice,' Renée admits 'but we corresponded weekly for many years.'

Clothilde's mouth drops open in astonishment.

'It was Camille that introduced me to the joys of literature,' Renée explains. 'Not just English literature mind, she loved our own French literature too, and she was also exploring works in Italian and even German.'

Clothilde stiffens at the memory that it was Camille's German language skills that had taken her to work in Vichy and had ultimately led to her disappearance. Luckily her aunt's reminiscing takes another turn, before Clothilde's distress reaches a level where she needs to make an excuse to leave the room.

'Camille of course had an equal passion for the visual arts,' Renée continues. 'Which I have to admit, I never shared, other than as an appreciation for beautiful clothes, and an elegant home.'

Renée gestures around the room.

'Your mother would keep me up to date by sending me articles that she had cut from magazines, handbills that had been given to her on the streets of Paris, and long, long letters, regaling me with all her experiences, penned in the most beautiful handwriting – it was almost calligraphy.'

Clothilde is holding her breath. Finally, she screws up the courage to ask.

'Do you still have the letters?'

Renée's face falls, and Clothilde wants to cry, as she can see the answer before her aunt speaks.

'Times were hard here during the war, and there was a moment when we had no way to light a fire during a terrible winter storm. I was re-reading one of the letters at the time, and I couldn't hold out when Jagu insisted that our ability to survive was dependent on getting that fire going. Of course, now I wish I had thought to tear pages from my books instead, but with the Nazi book burning of the 1930s, I had come to see books as sacrosanct.'

Clothilde nods her head. She can't really blame Renée. Her mother had written to her a few times from Vichy when she was a girl, and she hadn't thought to keep those communications either.

It is only now, in this moment, that the details of those childhood letters resurface, faint at first, the memories gradually coalesce. Whilst the communications had held the expected sentiments of a mother separated from her daughter, each one had also included a line from a children's poem, with a request that Clothilde find out which poem it was and then learn it.

Each time Clothilde would start with her grandparents, and then Rory and Dominique, but, if necessary, she would tour the whole village until she found someone, often an older student, who recognised the line and could teach her the poem. The faces of the villagers float in her mind's eye, she hasn't thought of these people, those poems, or her mother's letters for more than seven years. For the gift of these memories, she is immensely grateful.

Isla - 2018

It is totally maddening trying to piece together the story of Mam's life from these tiny fragments of information. I have so many questions and no one to ask. Did Mam ever write back to Renée? If she did, surely Renée would have mentioned it to her sister? Simone has confirmed that she herself wrote without hope of reply. It seems that Lorna was the only one for whom Mam broke her strict self-imposed silence.

I settle down to write to Adjavella. At least the sadness of the tale that I have to tell is counterbalanced by the vibrancy of the friendship between Lorna and my mother. The vision of the pair of them, running around the farms as little girls in wartime, brings joy to my heart. I hope perhaps one day Adjavella and Lorna can meet.

I know too, that Adjavella will understand the way that childhood instability can provide a background explanation for all sorts of psychological disorders. That my mother found a way to cope with her pain and give an outward appearance of normality - at least most of the time - is testament to her phenomenal strength.

Thank goodness that whilst there was so much loss in her early life, there was also love.

Unfortunately, it's clear that Mam's arrival here in Quiberon was not straight forward. I have been welcomed with open arms by my newly found family. I think that a younger generation, and changing times, have something to do with the warmth that I feel.

It is a huge shame that Mam was given into the hands of the wrong sister. Simone is a demonstrative person, and obviously warmed to Mam instantly. I can see that Mam would have easily settled into life on the farm at Kervihan.

Unfortunately, from the little that I have uncovered about my great aunt Renée, she sounds like an uptight woman, and not naturally given to the role of mother, especially to a spiky teenager.

Life with Renée would have been the opposite of what I would have needed, to feel safe and secure. But perhaps Mam would have mistrusted anyone asking her to be emotionally connected at that time. Maybe being fed and clothed in combination with a tiny room of her own, had been enough to allow her to find her own way.

Clothilde - 1956

Clothilde is sitting on the sheepskin on the floor in her room, looking out of the window across the fields to the wild coast. There are times when she stands on the cliff top and wonders about just letting go. But she knows she will never have the nerve to do it. Unfortunately, the courage to go on seems equally lacking.

Allowing herself to become so attached to James has been a mistake. He has made such progress with his rehabilitation over the last couple of weeks, that he will surely be announcing his departure any day now.

At which time, she will be back to a daily existence with no friends, and no real purpose in life. The thought of saying goodbye to him is unbearable, and she is simply not going to do it.

There have been many losses, but very few goodbyes in her life. She hadn't had a chance to speak to either of her parents before they were gone, and she had left it far too late to say goodbye to either of her grandparents. She'd been in denial each time, and they had both been too ill to understand what she was saying when she did finally speak. Therefore, her first real goodbyes were to the Stewarts and Olivier when she left Barantan.

Climbing into the train at Vichy had been almost impossible. She had wanted to cling to Rory, begging him to let her stay. Whilst at the same time, she had wanted to lash out, to punish him for sending her away. In the end, she had let the ice spread down her jaw, and throughout her body. Pecked them all on the cheeks and climbed into the carriage without a word. Merely waving from the window as the train set off.

She will not do another train station farewell.

Neven is making a trip this weekend to pick up some second-hand equipment from his cousin's farm near Sarzeau. He will be gone for three or four days. He doesn't know it yet, but she will be going with him.

Isla - 2018

Today Simone is in rather a lot of pain, so we've altered our plans. We are currently sitting in the car up on the headland with the doors open, drinking tea out of a thermos.

'It's nice to leave the house, especially after heavy rain. The air always smells so fresh.'

Simone has her head tipped back as she inhales deep lungfuls of Atlantic air.

'I'm glad it's worth the pain of getting into the car.'

'To be outside is always worth that. I spent my whole life outdoors, and this new arrangement at Philippe's makes me feel like I'm an exhibit in a museum.'

I let out a loud snort of laughter. It is appallingly easy to forget that elderly people are still vibrant, and full of humour on the inside.

'Renée's house is a little like a museum isn't it! How did you two sisters grow up to be so different?'

'Renée had a competitive personality, and when she met your grandmother, it triggered a need in her to be 'the best'. In her case that meant being the most up to date about social trends, or Paris fashions.'

Simone pulls a face, and I can see what she thinks of her sister's priorities in life.

'Are you similarly driven?' I ask, unsure of what really motivates my great-aunt.

'Luckily, I'm not in the least competitive. In fact, I'm rather happy if things stay the same. I like the stability that brings. I even liked that Neven and I carried on using animals to plough the fields and pull the cart, long after many farmers had bought tractors and other machinery.'

'But that must have been physically exhausting. Surely it wasn't worth it just to avoid change?' I remark incredulously.

However, once I say this, I remember my mother's stubborn streak. Perhaps Simone similarly dug her toes in, against all logical argument. But I'm soon to be enlightened.

'We had no money for new machinery, and as the other farmers in the area mechanised, they would give away the horse-drawn ploughs, scythes and other equipment they no longer had use for, so we were able to restock our farm at very little cost.'

I bob my head, acknowledging their financial logic.

'Reducing out-goings on repairs in this way kept us viable into the mid-sixties. By that time, we had saved enough money for a tractor and a Renault 4.'

The Renault 4 is such a classic small car. I've seen them transport everything from a musician with a double bass, to a family of five with all their luggage for a two-week holiday, so I'm not at all surprised to hear that one could also be used for live animal transport, and other farm related tasks.

'With these two new vehicles we were able to run the farm until the late seventies, but by then Neven, who was eight years older than me, had developed terrible arthritis, and could no longer conduct the heavy labouring the job requires. It was heart-breaking, but we sold off the land to housing developers, and retired on the proceeds.'

'My great-grandparents were about to face a similar decision in Barantan before Mam moved here. It was only ill health that took the decision from their hands.'

Once again, I'm filled with sadness that not a trace of their property had remained, after the developers had finished.

'That post-war period saw the end of small-scale farming all over France. Neven and I lasted longer than most.' Simone reflects.

'At least Odile still has your farmhouse.'

'Yes, for that I'm grateful. We were very happy there. I hate the idea of it being knocked down.'

'Why don't we drive on up there?' I suggest. 'If Odile is home we can go in, but if not, we can just sit outside, and you can tell me stories about your life.'

Simone beams with delight at the idea, so we pack up and get on our way.

As we pull up in the street outside the farmhouse, I'm about to get out and ring the doorbell, when Simone starts to speak.

'The last time I saw your father, during his 1956 convalescence, was a day just like today.'

My head snaps around in her direction.

'Oh, please tell me. I know so little about Da as a young man.'

'Well, he was very attractive, so it is no surprise that Clothilde fell for him, and he was also very kind and thoughtful. But completely impossible to understand!'

James - 1956

As James approaches Jagu Tangye's home, he begins to gnaw at a piece of loose skin at the edge of his thumbnail. Jagu does not approve of his relationship with Clothilde, and James is unsure of the reception he will receive.

However, he's desperate to speak to her, as he's not heard from her in three days, which is very unusual. Arrangements have finally been made for his return to Britain, and she needs to know.

He will be travelling by train on Monday morning to connect with the Night Ferry that will take him across the channel. They have one final weekend together and he wants to make the most of it.

For the last two days it has been raining solidly. The continuous downpour is perhaps a reason Clothilde might not have wanted to step outside. Although, it has never stopped her before. In fact, in the past, rainy days have always meant that they could spend a full day together, as she was not needed on the farm.

Today, with the last of the decorating jobs complete, James is free to seek her out, and so here he is. He knocks firmly on the door. It's eight o'clock in the morning, which is early to be calling, and he knows he is risking Jagu's wrath, but he doesn't want to miss any of their potential day together.

However, much to his surprise, it appears that no one is home. He walks around to the back of the house, where Jagu stores his fishing gear. It is all gone, so Jagu and Bernard must be out already.

Clothilde's bike is also missing, which suggests that she might be up at the farm. It's a further forty-five-minute walk to Kervihan, and it has already taken him twenty minutes to reach this point.

This is going to be the biggest endurance test of his leg to date, but he is determined to find her. Hopefully he will be able to share Clothilde's bike on the return journey.

The route looked different at walking pace, and there were a few times when he was forced to pause and retrace his steps, to be sure that he was on the right road, but the familiar names of Rue des Quatre Vents, the village of Kerné, the Rue de Kerniscob, and the hamlet of Kerboulevin have finally brought him limping into the farm, where he is greeted by Simone.

'James! Good morning! What are you doing here?' Simone's English is halting but proficient.

She seems both pleased, and oddly surprised to see him.

'I've come to see Clothilde.' James tries to speak clearly and reduce his regional accent as much as possible. He gestures towards Clothilde's bike, which is lying on the ground under the lean-to at the end of the barn, in the hope that Simone will make the connection. Although he would have thought it was obvious that his appearance here could only have one purpose.

'James, she's not here. She cycled up at first light. She and Neven left at 5am for the journey to Sarzeau.'

'Sarzeau? Where's that?'

With the crash of sudden disappointment, James is acutely aware that he needs to sit down and starts casting around for somewhere to rest.

Simone, understanding his predicament, invites him inside, and before long they are sitting at the kitchen table drinking coffee.

'James, they have gone to collect some farm equipment. They won't be back until Tuesday.'

'Tuesday! But I'm leaving on Monday morning!' James is completely heartbroken.

Isla - 2018

'Your father came to the farm early one morning having walked all the way from Renée's. He was searching for your mother, as it was his final weekend and he wanted to spend it with her.'

I smile indulgently.

'Were they very in love?'

'Yes, absolutely, and I had to watch his heart break, right there in front of me, because your mother had guessed that he would be leaving and had run away.'

I stare at Simone in disbelief.

'You mean she literally ran away?'

'No, she just couldn't face another separation, and had requested to accompany Neven on a trip that he was making. We hadn't realised the significance of the timing. Neven had been delighted at the idea of another pair of hands, so had said yes without thinking about it. Of course, afterwards, we both wished that he had said no.'

I can see the regret on her face even now.

'So, after all those months together, they never got to say goodbye?'

I can just imagine what this would have done to Da. He was never good with separation either, but in the opposite way, he liked to hold people close, and keep them happy.

'Couldn't Da have waited until she got back?'

'No, his trains and ferries were all booked. He had come up to the farm to tell her the news. I think it was the cruellest thing your mother ever did, and I include walking away from all of us a few years later. I do understand why she did it, but that young boy was utterly devastated.'

'But she couldn't have done it deliberately. You just said that he hadn't told her yet.'

'Clothilde had a sixth sense about people who were going to leave her or let her down. She might misunderstand people in all sorts of other ways, but without fail, she could sense someone who was about to become unreliable.'

'So, she avoided saying goodbye. But she didn't avoid the separation.' I point out. 'She must have been equally upset when she got back, and her fears were confirmed.'

Thinking of all Mam had experienced, I can barely imagine the pain she must have felt.

'There were no tears. I gave her the news the moment I saw her. I think part of me was reprimanding her for hurting James that way. But all she said was 'I knew he'd go,' and then she went back to unloading the cart.'

'That was it?'

'Yes, she spent much more time in her room for the following months, and barely spoke to any of us, but there were no tears, and she never once mentioned his name. It was eerie. She had been in a rather similar state when she first arrived in Brittany, but somehow this time it was more noticeable. Her withdrawal couldn't be put down to shyness in a new environment with new people, as we all knew exactly how outgoing and happy she had been during the previous months. We tried desperately to engage with her, but she wouldn't respond.'

Clothilde - 1956

The trouble with being the one left behind is that everywhere you go there are memories of the person who has gone. Clothilde is regretting having shown James so much of the peninsula, because she now has no sanctuary other than the chapel in Saint-Julien and her bedroom.

She has therefore been dividing her free time between the two. The rest of the house is also free of association, as James never actually came inside, but it is hard to put the required smile on her face for her aunt and uncle, and Bernard is a merciless tease whenever he sees her.

So, for now, Clothilde's world has shrunk to the space within these four tiny walls.

She has thought about using the time to write to Lorna, but thoughts of Lorna lead to memories of Rory, and memories of Rory all involve Scotland, and thoughts of Scotland bring her back to James, and to the knowledge of how much she misses them all, and that pain is unbearable.

Every time she opens her heart, she eventually ends up being dragged back into this whirlpool of pain, and there is one thing that she is certain about - she can't go through it again.

So, she is going to have to find a path in life that avoids connections with other people. Perhaps she should become a nun. It's not something she has ever considered before, but it would ensure her separation from others, and the chapel is a great source of comfort at the moment.

The only problem with this plan is that she isn't particularly religious. The building, the people in the congregation, and the links with the Auvergne are all extremely important to her, but she dare not actually believe in God, because if she did, she would be so angry with him for taking away all the people that she's loved.

Twenty-seven

<u>Isla -2018</u>

It's Friday evening and once again I am at Philippe's for dinner. This is my final weekend, for although I am retired, and could stay indefinitely, I only have the hire car until Sunday night, when I'm due to fly back to Germany.

In many ways it seems a shame to go so soon, when I have only just met everyone, and especially with Simone being so elderly, but they all have busy lives, and I don't want to outstay my welcome.

With this in mind, I want to be sure that I have followed every lead to my mother's past, and there is one that I wish to return to.

'Philippe, before I go, would it be possible to take one more look at your grandmother's letters? I know we were looking for correspondence from Camille last time, but might there also be something from my great-grandmother, Chloe? I know that she wrote a letter asking if Mam could come and live here. Or perhaps she wrote to you Simone?'

'No, Chloe definitely wrote to Renée. I remember her showing me the letter when it came. Do go up and check Philippe, it's not the kind of thing your grandmother would throw away.'

Whilst Philippe goes in search of the letter, I turn to Simone.

'Do you mind if we return to Mam and Da's story? How did they find their way back to each other? I mean, I know they did, because I wouldn't exist if they hadn't, but when we were up at Kervihan, you were telling me how Mam had let Da leave without saying goodbye.'

'Their reunion was so romantic. Your father licked his wounds for a few months and then he started writing her letters. He wrote one a month for a year. As far as I know the first few were what you would call love letters, but when he got no reply, he started to write to her about his life, just day to day stuff you might share with a friend.'

'She didn't write back?'

I can't believe my mother. Well actually I can, all too easily, imagine her doing this. I've been on the receiving end of exactly this kind of behaviour.

Simone tries to justify Mam's actions.

'She was thinking of becoming a nun, and romantic overtures from a young man didn't fit with that path in life.'

'A nun!'

I burst out laughing. I can't think of anyone less suitable for being a nun than my mother, she was many things, but piousness was not one of them.

'Eventually something in one of the letters prompted her to reply, and from that moment they corresponded regularly, until one day who should come walking up the path to the farmhouse - hat in hand - but James?'

'He came back?'

'He did indeed. In the spring of 1959, he crossed on a British boat to Jersey and then joined a French boat to St Malo. During the two and a half years he had spent back in Scotland, he had built on the French that Clothilde had taught him and had managed to put together a convincing enough tale of love and heartbreak. A string of soft-hearted French trawlermen brought him all the way around the coast to Port Maria!'

I feel a warmth spreading fiercely across my chest, at the idea of Da wearing his heart on his sleeve in such a way, especially in a foreign language. He was always a man of great heart, but usually of small gestures. This whole tale pays huge tribute to the love that he had for my mother.

Simone is keen to tell me the rest.

'He had gone to a lot of effort to look smart in a white shirt, and grey flannel trousers, he even had a trilby instead of his fisherman's cap. Of course, he had been travelling for several weeks, so everything was a little rumpled.' She smiles indulgently.

'But if he'd been travelling for so long, didn't his letters stop coming?'

I can't bear the idea that Mam would have been cross with him for not writing when he arrived. There have been so many times in my life when Mam found it hard to switch out of one mood and into another, even if something lovely was happening. It is all too easy for me to imagine it happening during this situation.

'Luckily James had thought of that and arranged for someone back in Scotland to gradually post a stack of letters that he had written in advance, so that she would receive one a week until he got here. Two or three arrived after he did!'

The smile spreading over Simone's face is one of deep joy from across the decades.

'So, she wasn't expecting him at all?'

'No, but she was out in the field when he arrived, and she ran to catch up with him before he reached the house. We saw it all out of the kitchen window. He had brought her a single orange rose and he went down on one knee and asked her to marry him, right on the same spot where I told him she had run away. It was so poignant.'

'Please tell me she said yes!' I am desperate for there to be no more pain in my father's story, but my mother's track record is not good.

'I think all her intensions to keep him at a distance were swamped by the strength of her feelings. She was so delighted to see him that she just broke down. She was crying and hugging him and somewhere along the way she obviously said yes, because that was what James told us when they eventually joined us in the farmhouse.'

'It sounds like Da had got to know her well. It was a good decision not to warn her he was coming.'

'I'm certain that if he had behaved any differently, she would never have said yes.' Simone agrees. 'Changing the tone of his letters to friendship, with enough time between them to remove any pressure, allowed her to start reading them properly. As soon as she did that, their connection was re-established. Any hint that he was about to visit would have terrified her. Even after all that time she was still keeping the rest of us at arm's length. It was almost like she had made a vow never to feel anything again.'

'So, Da turning up, out of the blue, burst the dam.'

'It did indeed. Neven and I were delighted. Renée and Jagu took a little more convincing, as they still thought James was too young. However, he was twenty-one by this time, and I reminded them that I had been considerably younger than Clothilde when I got married. Neven also pointed out that James had proven himself a more than capable young man, having shown such initiative in the way that he had returned to propose.

'Did Mam actually need anyone's permission to marry by this time?'

'Oh no, she was twenty-three and an independent woman in the eyes of the law, but she was still living with Renée and Jagu, and they were always going to have plenty to say on the matter. Luckily, they changed their minds fast enough to avoid a scene.'

Philippe returns to the kitchen carrying a fragile looking grey envelope.

'I think this is the one you're after.' He says, passing it across to me. 'I turn it over to see *Chloe Guery, Barantan* written on the back.

I delicately remove the letter from inside and spread it out on the table. It's written in a very spidery hand, which drifts across the page, unable to keep in a straight line. The tears spring to my eyes, for I know that Chloe was just days from death as she wrote it, with no energy to spare, and needing to make every word count.

Dear Madame Tangye,

I believe you are the sister of the late Henri Marec, the father of my granddaughter, Clothilde Marec.

She is currently fourteen years old and has been living with me, here in Barantan for the last ten years. Her mother disappeared when she was six, we presume her to be dead at the hands of the Germans. My husband died a few years ago and it is now clear that I am dying too.

When I am gone Clothilde will have no one. I beg you to take her in, or perhaps your sister could if you are unable to do so, although I believe she is not very much older than Clothilde.

Clothilde is a sad child, but she works hard every day for her family, and she has never given me any trouble. I am deeply fond of her, and I know that you too could love her if you got to know her.

I am asking my friend and neighbour to post this letter for me, and it is possible that I will be dead by the time you reply. Therefore, please address any correspondence to Rory Stewart, Barantan.
Yours in hope,
Chloe Guery.

Isla - 2018

My tears splash down onto the page, and I quickly brush them away. I can imagine Chloe, barely able to lift her head off the pillow, summoning the last ounces of her strength to write this final letter for Rory to post, and at the same time I can imagine Renée sitting next door, or here in this kitchen as she opens this letter that will change her life forever.

Simone is watching me, and I pass the letter towards her, until I remember that her eyesight is no longer up to reading.

'It's ok,' she says noticing my hesitation and the reason for it. 'I remember every word of that letter, but I wanted you to be able to read it for yourself. Your great-grandmother was a remarkable woman, wasn't she? To be able to write such a letter in her final hours.'

I still can't speak so I simply nod.

'Renée and I instantly agreed that Clothilde should come here. We had always wondered what had happened to Camille and her daughter after Henri died, but we had never had an address, other than the one in Paris. We had no idea where to start the search for them.'

This is news to me. I had always assumed that war had made long distance communication difficult, and that Henri's family hadn't been that interested in forging a relationship with Mam when she was a small child.

'Renée was devastated at the news of Camille's disappearance,' Simone continues, 'and for many years she actually held out hope that her friend might one day return, but in the meantime, she believed that having her daughter to care for was an honour.'

I almost choke with suppressed mirth at this. I suspect that the reality of taking in a withdrawn and rather sullen teenager with a very troubled past was rather different from the fantasy of caring for her beloved friend's daughter.

For whilst this attitude rings true in the context of what I've heard about Renée's relationship with Camille, it certainly doesn't correspond to what I've uncovered about her interactions with Mam.

'Simone, what do you think happened to Camille?'

Tonight, feels like my only chance to ask this question, which has been haunting me.

'From what Lorna told me, Chloe obviously thought her daughter was in the resistance and may have been discovered and killed for it. However, Joseph doesn't seem to have shared that opinion.'

'I may be being extremely uncharitable here, but on the few occasions that I met Camille, she struck me as incredibly self-centred and avaricious. From what I knew of her, and the issues she considered important in the letters that she wrote to Renée, she would not have enjoyed the privations of rationing.'

I'm shocked by this new perspective.

'I have to confess, that at the time it crossed my mind that she might have been a collaborator - many people were, especially in the area around Vichy - despite their absence from the history books. It's not a part of our past that we are proud of as a nation.'

Simone does indeed look filled with unease, but she continues.

'It was easy to imagine Camille getting involved with a Nazi officer who could offer her luxuries unavailable elsewhere. She loved Clothilde, but it had taken her a long time to accept the changes that a child brought to her life in Paris.'

'Oh no! Don't tell me Mam was unwanted even as a tiny baby?'

'Henri wrote us letters detailing the evenings and weekends during that first year, when he stayed at home with Clothilde, whilst Camille went out with her friends, or he pushed the pram in the park, whilst Camille remained at home in bed. The truth of the matter is that Camille took a long time to bond with Clothilde, and she had never intended to be a single parent.'

I sit back utterly stunned.

Twenty-eight

Isla - 2018

My hotel room is strewn with papers as I try to collate everything that I've learnt about my family. I started off making notes in my phone after each conversation, but the size of the device was infuriating, with such significant and complex events.

Even with the larger computer screen, it has still been difficult to see the connections. So, I have gone old school, and written each story on its own page.

I have placed information about Mam beside information about Da, because sometimes they're linked. But information about Henri and Camille has its own area, and I am currently working on what I know about Chloe and Joseph.

With every clue that I've found, something has been revealed of the life, or personality, of one of my family members, and each time it has caused me to question my understanding of myself.

For there can be no denying, that some of who I am will be the result of genetic inheritance or generational exposure to personality traits, from these slowly emerging people.

As the hours to my departure tick by, I am starting to realise the consequences of having an extended family. The sadness that is building, with the knowledge that I have to say goodbye to them all, is something that I've never known.

The idea that I belong with them, that I could have a place here, that they want me in their lives, means such a lot.

I'm unsure if this new sadness at separation is a product of the increased number of people that I'm leaving behind - each bond adding its pain to the total loss - or whether it is just that the nonchalant way that I used to say farewell to my parents, has been shown by grief, to be the action of ignorance.

I certainly never took time to imagine how I would feel if I never got to see them again, and now with Simone, it is all I can think about. So, I've arranged to spend all day with her tomorrow.

Tonight therefore, is my chance to say goodbye to Fabienne and Erwan.

I will especially miss Fabienne. The days that I've spent with her have been beautifully easy, and not just because she speaks wonderful English, which has been a huge relief to my overloaded brain.

She and I have discovered that we have a lot in common, and with only a few months separating us in age, our worldviews are remarkably similar. There is an added closeness too, from the subtle recognitions of family gesture, and shared features which make a cousin a truly wonderful thing.

As it is almost time for dinner, I start to pack for tomorrow. I fetch my portable document box from where it has been at the bottom of my large suitcase, out of sight and out of mind in the wardrobe.

As I open it, I catch sight of the original batch of letters from the secret compartment. Life has been so hectic with so many sources of new information that I somehow managed to forget that I'd brought them with me. I was so focused on waiting for Adjavella's translations.

I abandon the idea of packing, and instead, I use the remaining minutes, to assess whether my French has improved enough - after all this time talking daily with native speakers - to read them for myself.

Echoing my experiences in Philippe's house, I once again find myself overwhelmed by the experience of holding my great-aunts' own words in my hands. When I opened the bundle of letters in Andrew's kitchen, I hadn't known any of the individuals concerned, so the letters had merely been a source of intellectual curiosity.

Since I've been here in Brittany, some of the personalities have become real-life flesh-and-blood family. Through the letters that Philippe has shared with me, I have also come to feel deeply connected to those long dead.

I'm totally unprepared when halfway through the pile, I come across an envelope in my father's handwriting, addressed to Mam here in Brittany.

One of the letters that Simone was talking about!

I quickly flick through the remaining envelopes. Six are from Da.

Elspeth must have put them straight in the *done* pile when she saw that they were in English. I'd been in full flow, filling her in about everything I discovered in the Auvergne, and she had probably assumed that I knew they were there, so there was no need to mention it.

Careful not to rip the envelope in my haste, I prepare to enter my father's heart. As with the anniversary letters, I'm a little embarrassed at the thought of how personal they might be, but Simone's reassurance about the style of these communications rings in my head, so I begin to read.

Clothilde - 1959

Clothilde is sitting on the stone wall in the hay field. In her hand is a letter from James. When he first started writing to her, she was incredibly annoyed, as it interfered with her determination to forget him. So, she had put the first few letters straight in the fireplace, feeling a certain satisfaction at his inability to reach her, as she watched them go up in flames.

However, with the passing months, she has come to appreciate his value as a pen friend. She can tell him anything about her life here on the peninsula, and he is able to recognise the places and the people that she refers to, unlike Lorna who has never had the chance to meet this side of her family.

These days when the letters arrive, she waits until she can be alone, as now, to open them. She tears open the envelope in her hand, and to her delight James has once again filled the margin of his letter with little drawings.

It is unclear whether these are absent-minded doodles, or deliberate illustrations, but whatever they are, they are beautiful depictions of the animals and plants that he sees on the shore in his native Scotland. The letters themselves are always written on the paper that has been used previously to wrap his lunch, as they are regularly covered in grease spots, and every now and then the odd crumb makes its way into the envelope as well.

Apparently, he has returned to trawler fishing, which pays reasonably well, and he is in the process of saving for a small house, as he doesn't want to continue living with his parents. Not that he currently sees much of them, as he has little time ashore.

His leg has fully healed, but he admits to being a little worried about his shoulder. It twinges every now and then when he pulls at an odd angle, and he can feel a weakness that wasn't there before his accident. He dare not say anything to the rest of the crew, but he's worried about a repeat dislocation out at sea.

Clothilde feels surprisingly protective of her friend. The idea of him being injured again, is something she feels personally responsible to help him guard against, she must write back and encourage him to visit a doctor next time he's on shore.

She looks up from the page, trying her best to conjure up this land she has never seen, and the people that he talks about.

She blinks hard. Her imagination has produced an incredibly exact hallucination. Someone that looks just like James is walking across in front of her down the track towards the farm.

She shakes her head to make it go away, but nothing changes. She pinches herself and closes her eyes, but when she looks again, he is still there.

Stuffing his letter into her pocket, she runs towards the hallucination. The only way to get rid of it is to run through it and prove to herself that he isn't there.

She doesn't say anything as she approaches. Instead, she just puts her head down and charges towards his chest.

James - 1959

James is desperately nervous. During the last few weeks, he has been single-mindedly focussed on making it to his destination, with little thought of the reception that he would get on his arrival. Now that he is here, Clothilde's reaction is all that he can think of.

There is no denying the connection that he and Clothilde formed during his convalescence, and in her recent letters her language has reverted to the warm, easy communication style of the hours they spent together two years ago.

However, the manner in which she cut him off and the degree to which she guards her heart from pain, are both indicators of the potential disaster that could follow his actions today.

James hears the sound of running feet behind him and turns just in time to brace himself for the head-down charge of Clothilde, who is almost on top of him. With his strong leg behind him and his arms out, he manages to lean in and stay upright as they collide.

He places his hands on her shoulders and pushes her back a little way so that he can see her face. She appears completely shocked and bemused by their collision.

'Hello!' He manages with the small amount of air remaining in his lungs. 'That's not quite the greeting I was expecting. Have you turned into a goat while I've been away?' he can't keep the laugh from his voice. 'Are you ok?'

Clothilde is muttering something to herself as she presses her hand against his chest. Then more clearly, she adds.

'What are you doing here?'

This wasn't how James had planned it, but he only has one answer to her question. So, he drops down on one knee in front of her, and taking the single orange rose from where it has been nestling in his pocket, he holds it up towards her as he says.

'Clothilde Marec, will you marry me?'

Clothilde - 1959

Clothilde watches as the surprisingly solid hallucination that she has created in her mind, drops down in front of her, and proposes marriage with a beautiful orange rose - not a ring, because her subconscious knows that for her, love and family are represented by roses, not jewellery.

As this is all a hallucination, she decides to be honest about how she really feels, so taking the flower from his hand, and raising it to her nose to see whether imaginary flowers are scented, she happily answers.

'I will!'

James - 1959

James stands. Unable to hold his joy, he bends down and kisses her deeply.

Once again, he is taken aback by the surprise and confusion in her reaction.

'What's the matter?' he asks, concerned that his joy is about to turn to misery.

'You're actually here?' Clothilde gives him a penetrating stare.

'Yes!' he agrees.

'And you just asked me to marry you, and I said yes?' She continues, her head cocked to one side, staring at him as if she hadn't been part of the previous interaction.

'Yes, I did, and yes, you did. Is that ok?'

James feels almost as bewildered as Clothilde sounds.

There is a long pause during which neither of them moves or speaks, and then Clothilde throws her arms around his neck, and in a tumult of emotion cries,

'Yes, yes, most definitely yes!'

Isla - 2018

Sure enough, rather than romantic overtures, these letters are full of day-to-day events, and funny stories with my paternal grandparents and from Da's time on the trawler. It seems that my grandfather had a passion for shinty that I never knew about. Apparently, he was away from home most weekends during the season, training or playing matches.

It's a game that has always terrified me. The idea that it is desirable to wield a massive wooden stick at head height, with enormous force, has made it almost impossible for me to sit and watch the game.

Whilst the anecdotes are interesting, my attention is grabbed by the string of little drawings around the margins of each letter. They almost say more about Da than any of his words.

Amongst the images, I recognise the specific shell shapes of the crab species that we would find together in our local rock pools when I was growing up, and many of the plants that grow along the shore. I can also name each of the hills that he has so accurately captured, in his sketched contour of the skyline across the water on the Isle of Arran.

I wish that I had been more of a letter writer whilst I was living in Germany, perhaps Da would have done something similar for me.

Isla - 2018

I arrive at Fabienne's house in Saint Julien as the light is fading, and I am welcomed in, first to the kitchen where I greet Erwan, and then to the dining room because the meal is ready.

'I hope you don't mind, Rozenn has stayed in Brest this weekend, so it is just the three of us.' Fabienne apologises for her daughter.

'Of course not, I remember what it's like to be at university. There is so much going on and dropping it all to spend time with an aged cousin you've never even heard of is never going to be appealing to a twenty-year-old. Besides, she may be in Brittany, but the university is not exactly close.'

'I don't know about that. I go back and forth all the time. She really should have been here.' Erwan grumbles, obviously unhappy at his daughter's decision.

'But you work from home most of the time, and even then, you stay in staff accommodation a few nights a week.' Fabienne points out.

'Seriously, it's ok,' I hastily add, before this conversation turns into a family dispute, 'She and I have met, and I'm sure we will have the chance to do so again. Perhaps she will come to Germany some time and I can show her around.'

'Oh, what a shame, I'd forgotten you live in Germany,' Erwan chips in. 'I've had it in my mind you were still in Scotland, with all the talk of your parents during the last few days. I was going to suggest that you look Nolwenn up when you got back.'

'Nolwenn's in Scotland?' I can't believe I missed this.

'Yes, she's been studying at Glasgow University for a while now.' Erwan confirms.

'Like Rozenn she wanted to explore her heritage, so she's doing an MA there, in Music and Celtic studies.' Fabienne elaborates.

'Glasgow! An hour away from Mam and Da.'

This revelation seems so unfair.

'And we never knew.'

My eyes fill with tears. I'm not sure what happened to the cut-throat businesswoman who never showed emotion. I seem to cry all the time these days!

'I agree,' Fabienne reaches out a hand to cover mine in support. 'If only we had all known. She would have loved to meet your parents. Unlike Rozenn, Nolwenn is very into family.'

'I feel a bit of a hypocrite being so upset,' I confess. 'I wasn't into family at all when I thought it was just Mam, Da and me. Ask anyone. I was a complete workaholic, hardly ever at home in Germany, let alone back in Scotland. But now that I've discovered all of you, I really regret that we never had the chance to spend time together.'

Isla - 2018

Last night's farewells were difficult but made easier by Fabienne's promise to try and organise a trip to visit me. This afternoon is so much harder because Simone is looking frail today.

Perhaps I've exhausted her with all my visits and questions, or maybe it's her own sadness at this parting, which might echo my mother's departure. Whatever the reason, we are standing beside my car holding hands, neither one of us wanting to be the one to say goodbye.

Odile comes to our rescue as she joins us on the street.

'Maman, this departure is different.'

She has obviously had the same thought as me.

'Clothilde warned us that she was making a clean break. Isla is doing the opposite. She has promised to come back as soon as she can, and whilst I know that you're not that keen on computers, I can help you have the occasional video call so that you can see where Isla lives and find out how she's doing.'

I nod enthusiastically.

'Oh, I'd like that.' Simone squeezes my hand tightly and looks deep into my eyes. 'I'm so delighted that you came to find us! It's like having your mother back in my life again, with all the memories that you've brought to the surface, and of course, you have her eyes. Did you know that?'

Twenty-nine

Isla - 2018

I've been home in Germany for six weeks now, and already I'm back in the office, working on a short consultancy project. The hours are not full time, and the demands are nothing in comparison to my previous job.

When I made the decision to retire, I was concerned that I would come to view it as a mistake. I was worried that losing my career, at the same time as both my parents, would feel like a third bereavement.

My life is certainly more mundane, but this has allowed me to grieve the loss of my parents in my own brittle way, away from the spotlight of my colleagues' gaze, and I am relieved that I don't regret my decision at all.

The biggest gift of retirement has been the discovery, through family, of a softer, more open side to myself, that seems totally incapable of staying away from my newly found relatives. Tomorrow I'm returning to Scotland, and this time, I will be introducing two new family members to the place we called home.

Fabienne is due to arrive at Glasgow airport soon after me. There we join up with Nolwenn, before travelling on to West Kilbride. I'm sad, that with the property sold, I can't take my cousins to stay in my parents' house, but we have found an Airbnb cottage near the Barony Centre, which looks very comfortable for three single adults, and I'm looking forward to showing them all the local places where I spent my childhood.

Isla - 2018

We are walking down the hill through the village, wrapped up against the October winds, but thankful that the day is dry.

'I know this may seem a little grim, but the first place I want to take you is the golf course where my father died. I want to pay my respects, but it's also a beautiful spot. You can see the Isle of Arran across the water, and it leads straight down to the beach. You get there on a footpath that leads past a cute little garden. It was one of Mam's favourite spots, even when her memory was going.'

Hearing myself talking about death and dementia in this way I realise how off-putting it must be to my new-found cousin. Nolwenn is a lovely young woman. She is dark-haired and petite, just like her mother, and I was very touched by the warmth of her greeting at the airport, as if we had known each other for many years, as opposed to never before.

Her English is very good and, as she replies to me now, I can hear that her accent is even developing a nice little Scottish inflection, as a result of the time she is spending in Glasgow.

'Wherever you take us is fine,' she says. 'It's all new to us. Any memory you share will help us get to know you, and Clothilde and James.'

A year ago, I couldn't have dreamed that I would find other people who would care about the lives of my deceased parents.

'I was so torn this summer when I heard that you were in Quiberon. I wanted to join you all, but I was at an incredible summer school in Ireland, and I didn't want to leave.'

'You had no way of knowing that I was going to suddenly show up out of nowhere.'

I'm distressed that she's been feeling guilty.

'Well, that's true, but I'm sad to have missed your first moments with the family.'

Nolwenn smiles compassionately at me, and my heart flips. For the first time in my life, I wonder what it would have been like to have a daughter.

Tilly - 2015

Tilly is both resting against the fence and leaning up against James for support. She can't understand why the simple act of standing upright seems so difficult these days. Her walking is slower too. In fact, lots of things are slower.

Like right now, she is looking at the little hump-backed bridge across the stream, and in the distance, to the left of the steps, she can see the plant with the long sword-like leaves and the red flowers.

Can she find the name for it? Absolutely not. She has been trying for at least the last five minutes, and yet she has known its name for many years, because they have one in their own garden.

This inability to find the word she wants is happening a lot, and more worryingly, yesterday when she was in the supermarket, she couldn't work out which coins to handover for her shopping.

At first, she hadn't recognised the currency, and then when she heard the shop assistant mention pounds, and not francs, she hadn't been able to do the maths to hand over the correct coins. In the end she had paid with a ten-pound note, just to be sure she was offering enough to cover her purchases.

As far as she's aware James hasn't noticed anything. He's always liked it when she holds his hand, or takes his arm, so he has welcomed the extra physical contact without questioning it.

The idea that she might be losing her memory or that something might be wrong with the rest of her body, like motor-neurone disease or multiple sclerosis, terrifies her.

And she's not only worried for herself. She and James have been together for almost sixty years. Their roles are given, and between them they are strong, but one can't work without the other.

James is so often away in his own head. He has no space in his mind for practical things like shopping and cooking so that he can eat, or doing the washing so that he will have clean clothes to wear.

Meanwhile the opposite is true for her. These day-to-day tasks are a major part of how she keeps herself calm. Routines and predictable events give her comfort. James oversees all the variable elements of their life. The tax return for the fish shop. The parent teacher meetings at the school. Hang on a minute. There haven't been any parent teacher meetings for decades. Isla left school in 1982.

Now she really is in a muddle. How could she not remember that Isla has left home? Especially when she has chosen to live in that awful country.

Isla - 2018

Our second stop of the day is Portencross Castle.

'It looks very old.' Fabienne says as she stares up at the boxed sides of the rather ugly tower.

'There's been a building on this site to provide defence since at least the mid-1300s. Although it's not always been this one.' I explain.

'Ooh, that's a long time!'

Nolwenn's interest has been piqued and she takes the information booklet from her mother.

'One of the things I love about studying here in Scotland is how many historic buildings survive to tell the stories of the generations gone by. All around us, in the landscape, but also in the folk tales. We can only truly make sense of who we are if we understand who our forebears were.' Nolwenn continues enthusiastically.

'There speaks a true historian!' Fabienne teases her daughter. 'Not everyone is as interested in the past as you and your father. The pair of you are lucky to know so much about the Gallon family. Don't forget, not everyone is able to trace their family back in time.'

'You know that was almost true for me?' I admit.

'Really, you mean you might not have found us?' Nolwenn seems touchingly distressed by this idea.

'Well, neither of my parents told me that Mam had cousins. I knew that neither of them had any siblings, so I had assumed that, as my grandparents were all dead, my parents and I were the last of my family.'

'So, how did you find out that we all exist?' Nolwenn asks, sitting down on the wall that separates the castle from the sea.

I take a seat beside her as I continue.

'If Mam had had her way, I would never have known about her past. But little clues kept popping out, because of her dementia. She couldn't keep her secrets straight in her mind. I genuinely had no idea what was going on. The things she was saying didn't make any sense when put together with the information that I'd always been given.'

'But why did she hate our family so much that she wanted to keep us apart?'

'Oh Nolwenn, she didn't hate us.' Fabienne quickly jumps in. 'She just wanted a fresh start. I know that's hard to understand. Especially for those of us to who have lived through peaceful times, but Clothilde's mind was full of unspeakable things that happened during the war.'

'But the war was such a long time ago.' Nolwenn points out. 'If she hadn't made that decision, we could have all met up and had a wonderful time when I first moved here. Surely seventy years is long enough to forget.'

'Unfortunately,' I say, sadly 'the war years eventually became all that she could remember.'

Tilly - 1969

Tilly and James are spending a rare evening out. The first in five years. They have organised for Isla to spend the night with a friend from her class. Tilly is anxious but James is so excited about the party.

Two young lads from the trawlers have recently become engaged and have been granted permission to have a joint celebration in the grounds of the castle.

It's nothing fancy. Just a beer keg by the harbour and Callum's Mam frying sausages over a fire that she's built in a cleft in the rock. Two of Hamish's mates are playing guitars and singing, and people are dancing in the grass.

This is the first time that James and Tilly have been out for an evening since Isla was born, but she hasn't minded. The evenings at home are her favourite time of day. Alone with James, once Isla goes to sleep.

However, she knows that James has been very keen to be out and about with her again. He's been very patient with her reluctance.

It's not being away from home, or leaving Isla, or even being in the open air that she minds. It's the need to be amongst other people that she finds hard. Risking their judgment, opening herself up to being shunned. She has sworn to do everything in her power to prevent that happening again.

She's worked hard to ensure that her accent is as similar to James' as she can manage, and she's not told a soul in the village where she's from. She has made James swear an oath of secrecy, and so far, no one has guessed that she is not from somewhere in Scotland.

She has a few acquaintances in the village, and now that Isla is at school, she even has a couple of women that she would call friends, but for the first four years living here in West Kilbride, it was her parents-in-law that formed the daily building blocks of her social life.

Now that they have retired and moved over to Arran, life in West Kilbride has become a lot quieter.

All week, James has been insisting that the benefit of coming along tonight, is the chance to meet other people from the village in a relaxed way. He wants her to chat and see whether there are people she might like to ask around for tea, or for a picnic on the beach if that seems too formal. Right now, she can't think of anything worse, but at least she's here.

Isla - 2018

As we walk on, leaving the immediate surroundings of the castle, I continue my story.

'Mam and Da used to bring me here when I was a child, and I would play in the grass, and down at the harbour. Da worked on one of the boats that was moored here when I was very little, but by the time I was at school he had set up the fishmongers back in the village. The family who owned the boat used to use the cellars of the castle to store and repair their nets, especially in winter.'

'It's such a sweet little harbour. It's a fraction the size of Port Maria!' Fabienne comments.

'As you say, just a handful of boats really, and of course these days they're all pleasure boats.'

'So, the bit I still don't understand is how no one spotted that Tilly was French from her accent?' Nolwenn says, with a wrinkle between her brows.

'Well, as you and your sister are living proof, this family is full of great linguists.' Fabienne points out. 'I mean you are both fluent in Breton and French and speak excellent English, as well as the Gaelic you're learning now, and Rozenn's got Spanish and Welsh too.'

'Yes, but we were brought up bilingual as children, and have spent hours studying the other languages.'

'That's just it. Even though she lived in the Auvergne, Mam was brought up bilingual, by a Scot, and Fabienne's right, Mam had a gift for languages, passed down on both sides of her family. According to Simone, Henri spoke French, German and English well, along with some Flemish, Dutch and Italian and I know that Camille spoke excellent German as well as French, because it's what got her killed.'

'Seriously!' Nolwenn is shocked.

'Well actually I don't know that for sure. She was working as a translator in Vichy during the war and disappeared.'

'That's awful. Wow. I'm starting to understand Clothilde's torment.' Nolwenn looks apologetic.

Camille - 1941

Camille is sitting upright against the pillows of the bed, in the room that she shares with her daughter. Clothilde is snuggled up into her armpit, holding on tight to the arm that envelops her.

The afternoon sunlight is falling through the window directly onto her lap, and they are reading the copy of Erich Kastner's 'Emil and the Detectives' that Henri gave to her several years ago as one of her first German translation exercises.

If her father finds out that she has a German book in the house, he will probably throw her out. But Kastner was a pacifist, and the book was written for children. It also happens to be one of only a handful of items that she still has, that connect her to Henri, now that he is dead.

For she is certain that the landlord of their apartment building will have sold everything in lieu of unpaid rent by the time that she and Clothilde return. If indeed they ever get the chance to go back to Paris.

Clothilde - 1941

Clothilde is interested in the story that her mother is reading, partly because the boy in the story seems a little bit like her. His father is dead, and he is alone without his mother during most of the story. However, what is holding her attention the most is a fascination that her mother can read words in one language, and speak them aloud to her in a different one.

Although she is now able to speak quite a lot of English, thanks to Rory and Lorna, she still finds it difficult to swap from English to French. In fact, there are many things she can only say, and actually even think, in one language or the other.

However, what she likes most about them reading this book together is that she has her mother all to herself. Every time they read another chapter, she gets to lie in her mother's arms and breathe in her scent, as she listens to her favourite sound in the whole world - her mother's voice.

They have only got a few more minutes, because it is Sunday afternoon, and her mother must be back in Vichy by dark. It's horrible. The thought of her leaving always spoils the happiest bit of her visit.

Clothilde reaches her free arm across her mother's waist and squeezes her very, very hard.

Isla - 2018

Lunch today at the Seamill Hydro was really special, particularly after I explained that we had been due to celebrate my parents' wedding anniversary there a year earlier. We ended up having champagne and toasting them and their long and happy life together.

So, I'm now feeling more than a little tipsy as we walk back up the hill. I don't make a habit of drinking during the day, and it has gone straight to my head.

'Oh, Nolwenn look, how sweet, it's a letterbox. Look, it's almost completely hidden in this ivy.' I think Fabienne is as drunk as I am.

'I used to love posting my letters here as a child,' I say trying to stop her stepping back off the narrow pavement into the on-coming traffic as she admires her find. 'It somehow always seemed extra special, as if the letters would receive some magical assistance to reach their destination.'

Almost at once Fabienne has forgotten the post box and has another urgent thought.

'I've eaten too much, and this hill is very steep, is there anywhere we can sit down for a rest?'

'Sure.' I say with a smile. 'Just up here on the right there are some benches at the memorial. We can rest there for a while.'

The memorial, in my opinion, has been built at an odd spot. It's at the site of a four-way junction, on one of the busiest roads in the village.

'Mam used to come here all the time. I never really understood her choice, as West Kilbride is full of little gardens and parks with benches that would have provided much more peaceful spots for contemplation.'

Fabienne seems to be glad of the opportunity for a rest.

'Now that I know more about Mam's life, I wonder if she came here to think of her parents. After all, they were lost in the Second World War, and Rory Stewart fought in the First World War. They have no specific connection to this particular memorial, but it would have been a suitable place to come and remember them.'

'That seems very likely,' Nolwenn agrees.

As this is our last day together, I want to stop into the Barony Centre to buy some Scottish gifts for Simone and the others back in Quiberon. I leave Fabienne and Nolwenn looking around this week's exhibition and head over to the shop.

I'd love to buy some of the local pottery, but it would be heavy, and I don't want Fabienne to have to worry about it breaking during the flight. In the end I find some beautiful fingerless gloves for Simone. I hope that they will keep her joints warm, as she experiences a lot of pain in her wrists and hands.

For Odile I've found a pair of locally made earrings, and for Philippe some fisherman's socks to wear inside his boots when he is out at work. Erwan and Rozenn are a little harder, as I didn't have a chance to get to know them so well. But then I remember their love of history, and traditional ways of life, and I find a couple of small books about the local area which I'm sure will be right up their street.

This is such a new experience for me, shopping for gifts for family members. I've watched other people do it every year, at Christmas time and other festivals, and I've never realised how hard it is, but also how much fun.

I wonder what it must be like to have a room packed full of family and friends all there to celebrate with you. It's something I've never had. Christmas was always just the three of us, except when I was tiny, when I think Da's parents joined us, but I don't really remember.

On my birthdays I was allowed up to three friends for tea, because that was the number of spare chairs we had. And whilst I could have organised my own birthday parties as an adult, I never had much of a social life, and was always too busy at work to bother acknowledging another year gone by.

I can feel something brewing in my chest, and then in an excited rush the idea becomes fully formed. I can't wait to share it with the others. I drop my items on the counter next to the sales assistant. Much to her surprise I rush off, calling over my shoulder.

'Can I just leave those there for a moment?'

Panting slightly, from excitement rather than exertion I blurt out my idea.

'Fabienne, you and I are turning fifty-five this year, and Odile is going to be seventy. I think we should have a big party in France to celebrate it all.'

'Oh, what a brilliant idea. Do it in the holidays, then Rozenn and I can be there too!'

Nolwenn seems almost as excited as I am.

'I'm not sure that being fifty-five is much to celebrate,' Fabienne mutters.

'Oh, come on' I wheedle, nudging her shoulder with mine. It will be fun. I've never had a birthday party.'

'What, never?' Nolwenn is shocked.

'No, just small meals or outings. I've never really known enough people.'

'Well in that case we must do it.' Fabienne concedes. 'It will be a pleasure to host the best party you've ever had!'

'Not much of a challenge there, as it will be the only party she's ever had.' Nolwenn chuckles.

Thirty

Isla - 2018

After a week sharing a house with my cousins, my apartment has never felt so lonely. Far from being irritated by their proximity - which had been a concern of mine when I booked us into the Airbnb instead of individual hotel rooms - I had embraced the fun of staying up late with Fabienne and drinking herbal tea in our pyjamas curled up on the sofa, and of having people to eat toast with, in the morning.

The consultancy work is nearly finished. I'm not sure what is going to be next for me. Either I need the company to give me another project that hopefully requires a deeper commitment and is more of a mental challenge, or I need to do something to increase my connection to other people, because knocking around in this apartment on my own, with little to occupy my mind, is not healthy for me.

My trip back to West Kilbride has brought my parents to the front of my mind. I really miss them both, but Da particularly. I've been so absorbed in Mam's life for the last few months, that he has only appeared as a minor character on the periphery of my thoughts.

To bring him nearer to me, I decide to create a little exhibition of his watercolours around my living room. I fetch his bundle of letters from its place of safe keeping, in the box under my bed. Careful to pencil matching numbers on each letter and painting, I separate them out into a stack of letters and a long string of paintings on the rug in the middle of the room.

The Balloch waterfront with the steamer is followed by the view from Balmaha. Another of Balloch Castle and gardens - that I now realise I watched him paint when I was six - is followed by a view from the ridge above Arrochar. Then comes the beachfront at Luss, where I remember playing cricket with Da, and another of Rossdhu House.

I feel so lucky to have these paintings. Each one brings back a happy memory of a family occasion. In addition to being beautiful in its own right. With a further five paintings of the highlands and islands, and a few of the West Kilbride area spread out before me, I'm starting to wonder about asking the Barony Centre if they would be interested in having the pictures as part of a short exhibition. After all, Da was a local artist, even if he kept that secret from everyone except Mam.

I think it would be wonderful to acknowledge his talent, even if he's not around to see it. The only problem might be that none of them would be for sale, as I'm not prepared to part with them.

There are also three older pencil sketches, drawn on what seem to be blank pages that he's torn from books.

Now that I have been to the area, I recognise these as drawings done during his convalescence in Quiberon, or perhaps when he returned to ask Mam to marry him.

One is clearly the harbour at Port Maria, and another shows the standing stones at Kerbourgnec, but the last one I don't recognise, although it looks as if it is somewhere along the Atlantic coast of the peninsula, as I recognise the vegetation. I wonder how it escaped the list of places that I was taken to. It looks stunning.

The picture is of an amazing arch, carved out of the cliff by the sea. Perhaps, since the drawing was completed, erosion has caused it to collapse into the water. After all, it is approximately sixty years since Da drew this picture. I cross the room and put this sketch on the shelf beside Mam's ashes. I must remember to ask Simone about it when we video chat on Sunday.

Isla - 2018

I can see Odile and Simone sitting at the kitchen table. Philippe is wandering around in the background making a cup of coffee. Although this is the fourth time that we've done this, Simone is still a little confused by the whole process and distracted by her own image.

Hoping to pull her focus, I ask about the arch.

'Simone, I found this pencil sketch of my father's. I don't think you'll be able to see it when I hold it up to the camera, but perhaps I can describe it to you.'

'It's of an arch that's been warn into the cliff. Do you know where that would be?'

Simone replies immediately.

'Oh, that's the 'Arche de Port Blanc'. It's at the top end of the peninsula, about four kilometres from the isthmus.'

'You mean it's still there?'

'Oh absolutely, it's a wonderful place.' Odile nods enthusiastically.

I feel quite peeved. If it's such a wonderful place, why didn't they take me there?

'Unfortunately, I can't get there anymore,' Simone explains. 'There's a substantial walk to the cliffs from the car park and then a very steep decent down to the beach.'

'Oh, I see. That's a shame. It looks really beautiful.'

'It is. That's why it was chosen as the location for your parents wedding reception.' Odile adds.

I'm stunned at her words.

'Wedding reception?'

'After your parents' marriage at the Mairie in Quiberon, they drove the horse and cart up to the Arch. Maman and I had decorated it especially for them. I remember it so clearly. I was nine years old, and it was the first wedding I had been involved with.' Odile's eyes are shining as she describes it. 'We got reams of white satin and pinned it to the cart, with lots of pillows underneath to make it extra comfortable.'

Simone is nodding along and takes up the story.

'We created bouquets of roses and wildflowers from the garden at the farm and tied them around the cart. It looked so beautiful. The rest of us followed in a great procession all the way to the arch, where we had a huge celebration on the beach. It was a glorious day, topped off with a beautiful sunset. We stood watching it for ages from the headland.'

Clothilde - 1958

Clothilde and James are standing on the steps of the Mairie waiting for the big surprise. Odile has been practically exploding with excitement for the last week, and Simone has had to shush her twice this morning when she was about to let something slip.

As bride and groom, they have been deeply involved in the planning of the wedding up until this point, but Simone and Neven asked if they could make the reception a wedding gift. The details have been kept a complete surprise. All they know is that tonight they will be taken to a hotel in St Pierre Quiberon for a few nights mini honeymoon, thanks to Renée and Jagu.

Clothilde is deeply aware that for herself, and all her family members, this wedding is bittersweet. For it is both a celebration, and the gateway to their separation, which may have prompted the substantial generosity from both her aunts.

She knows that they disagree with her decision. But opportunities like this for a clean break and a cleansing of the mind, do not come along often, and nothing that she has tried over the last decade or more has had any impact on her inner distress. Nothing that is, until she met James.

Clothilde looks up at her husband. Mrs Clothilde MacLeod. It feels wonderful. But it doesn't sound quite right. Clothilde Marec was French. With her upcoming move to Britain, perhaps it's time for a fresh start.

Tilde MacLeod sounds more Scottish. She will need to register her change of last name, perhaps she can also legally replace Clothilde with Tilde. It would be marvellous to say goodbye to the name Clothilde forever and leave all the sadness with it in the past.

James - 1958

James is gazing down at his beautiful wife. Wife! She said yes! She didn't run away at the last minute! He'd been worrying for weeks that she wouldn't show up today.

It's been such a complicated process. There have been so many hurdles and they've both been deeply frustrated by the number of legal hoops they've had to jump through for the French authorities.

And it's not over yet, as they will need to go through the whole thing again once they arrive in Britain, but it's worth it. He now has the most beautiful, wonderful wife. They have a future, and whatever happens, they are going to be together.

James leans down and kisses Clothilde. The moment is broken by the sound of hooves on the road beside them, and they turn to see Simone driving the horse and cart with a beaming Odile sitting up front beside her.

The whole vehicle is completely transformed into the most beautiful wedding carriage. They pull up beside them and Odile jumps out to hold the horse's head.

Simone steps down and approaches her niece.

'Your carriage awaits, my dear.' She says with a sweeping gesture. 'It's a little unconventional, but I think we'll have you driving. James might have you overturned in a ditch along the way.'

Clothilde snorts with laughter and squeezes her new husband's hand as she steps forward towards the cart.

'That's fine, but where am I going?' she asks.

'To the arch! It's all planned!' Odile jumps up and down, she's so excited to finally be able to share her secret.

Clothilde - 1958

Clothilde and James are almost at the arch. She turns to look over her shoulder at the contour of the coastline leading south towards Quiberon and is stunned to see a stream of other vehicles processing behind them.

She had been aware that Jagu and Renée were following in his truck, with Bernard, Simone and Odile squashed in the back. But along the way from the mairie, various friends have also fallen in behind, to make up a string of about twenty vehicles.

Two of their farmer friends are also in horse-drawn carts, but most of the guests are driving trucks or cars, apart from a few teenagers on bicycles.

They all pull into the parking area. Neven and the other farmers remove the horses from the shafts and tether them to graze. It is then a case of *many hands make light work* as the other carts are unloaded. They have food and drinks, blankets, a couple of tables and a few folding chairs for older guests. These are now all heading for the beach.

Bernard taps James on the shoulder.

'Can I steal the two of you for a minute? I've borrowed a camera, and I want to take a few photographs on the headland before we go down and join the others.'

Clothilde is a little hesitant. She doesn't really like having her picture taken.

'Come on, you can't have a wedding without a photograph,' Bernard points out 'and anyway it will give the others a chance to set everything up just the way they want it, before the two of you go down there.'

Isla - 2018

I am delighted to learn that Mam got married in Quiberon, just like her parents. I hope she knew. It's wonderful, that after so much sadness in her life, she and Da got a perfect wedding day that they could cherish.

I can feel my cheeks starting to ache from smiling so much.

I reach up to replace the drawing on the shelf above my computer, next to Mam's ashes, and they spark an idea.

'Odile, I think I've finally decided what I would like to do with Mam's ashes. I want to bring her back and reunite her with all of you.'

Simone's head snaps upright and she is finally looking directly into the camera.

'If I pack her ashes when I come over for our birthday party, we could scatter her into the sea with all of us there to say goodbye. I would really like to take her back to where she was on her wedding day. It was obviously such a happy time. I know that Simone said that she can't walk out to the arch anymore, but might we be able to hire a beach-buggy of some kind to take her from the car park to the cliff top?'

Philippe leans over his cousin's shoulder so that he can look directly into the camera.

'I think that's a wonderful idea. I've got a friend I can ask. I'll make it happen. Now that Clothilde's mental health is no longer the issue, she should be back here with her family.'

Having come up with this plan for Mam's ashes there are a couple of very important people I need to contact.

First, I pick up the telephone.

'Lorna, is that you?'

'Isla, how lovely! Where are you, my dear?'

'I'm back in Germany, but I have a plan for us to possibly see each other again. How are you with travel these days? Might you be able to make it to Brittany on 6th June for a birthday party? My cousins and I are having a celebration of 180 years. Fifty-five of them are mine.'

'Just listen to the natural way you speak about your family! I'm so happy for you!'

I can feel her warmth oozing down the phone and I feel terrible. I've been so out of touch during the last few months. I'd promised myself I would be in regular contact with Lorna. But after a first flurry of activity, I've only sent a couple of emails in recent months. The insular habits of a lifetime need to be ditched!

'I'm sorry Lorna, there's no excuse. I should have been in touch.'

'Nonsense, life is busy, and in your case exciting! Anyway, you're calling me now, and that makes me happy. What's your plan? I'd love to be there.'

'I can't wait to meet Simone. I want to hear what happened to Clothilde after she left me.'

'I'm so excited to bring the two of you together.'

'I'm delighted to be invited!'

I can hear the excitement in her voice, and I equally can't wait to see her.

'There's another reason I was hoping you could come. I'm going to bring Mam's ashes and I want us all to be there to say goodbye together. You're a part of this big family too, you were Mam's foster sister during her time in Barantan. My relatives need to hear your memories. I want them to understand that you were her first family.'

There is silence for a little while and I'm worried that I might have said something wrong, but then Lorna speaks, and I can hear the lump in her throat.

'I love the idea that Clothilde has a huge family, that all want to get together to remember and celebrate the wonderful, adventurous, funny, anxious, isolated child that she was.'

'We definitely need more stories about that funny side. I've not heard much about it so far. Would you be willing to say a few words at the scattering?'

'I'll do my best. It will be an emotional day.'

The next person that I contact is Adjavella. I'm not sure where she's working now, or what shift she might be on, so I start with an email invitation to the party, and an offer to cover all her travel expenses, lost wages, and pay for an agency carer to cover any shifts she might miss, so that there can be no objections from her employers.

I want her to be able to see where Mam lived and meet all the people who knew her. The two of them had such a close relationship at Suncrest, Adjavella needs to be able to say goodbye with us.

Thirty-one

Isla - 2019

Philippe is hosting the party, with the help of outside caterers, and we have made a special arrangement to pitch a marquee on the piece of disused land across the road from the house. The company laid a wooden floor this morning, and later tonight a friend of Rozenn will function as DJ so that anyone who wants to, can dance.

Lorna and Simone are both threatening to do so, but they are currently holed up in Simone's room, swapping stories and reminiscing about Mam. I want to hear what they're saying, but this is my party, my first ever party, and I want to enjoy it.

Adjavella arrived this afternoon and is currently beside me chatting with Nolwenn about Glasgow. I'm sticking around to make sure that she's ok, as it's hard when you don't know anyone.

What am I thinking? It's hard for *me* when I don't know anyone. Adjavella, on the other hand is constantly starting work in new situations. She's used to talking to strangers, and her French is far better than mine. What am I worrying about?

I guess this anxiety comes with being a host for a social gathering. Things seem to be going well. The living room is packed with Odile's friends, all drinking wine and commenting about how much she's been missed at work.

Rozenn has invited several younger people of her own age, and they are lying on the grass around the marquee, drinking beer and listening to their DJ friend playing tracks that are too mellow for the dancing later.

With no separate group of friends of my own, I have stuck like glue to Fabienne. The four of us are standing in the street outside the kitchen door, directing late arrivals to the marquee, and available should the caterers need anything. At some point, I must force myself to go inside and mingle. That is, after all, the point of a party.

Fabienne breaks away from our little group and walks down the road with her arms outstretched towards a cluster of people.

'Ah, at last, you've arrived. Now the party can begin!'

She ushers them back up the street and stops in front of me.

'Everyone, I want you to meet my wonderful, newfound cousin Isla, and her friend Adjavella, without who's help Isla and I would never have met!'

Isla - 2019

Last night was a huge success. The marquee had been packed with people of all ages. Simone did dance to one track with Odile on one side for support, and Philippe on the other. However, she took herself off to bed at nine-thirty with strict instructions to us all to have fun on her behalf.

I'm feeling a bit woolly headed now as a result, but thankfully I stopped drinking well before midnight as I've got to drive the others up to the arch this morning. The rest of the family will be going direct and are meeting us there at 11am.

I head to the lobby and spot Lorna and Adjavella deep in conversation. They both look beautiful to say goodbye to Mam. Adjavella is wearing a traditional Senegalese outfit in a vibrant turquoise-and-blue print. She is attracting a lot of attention from the other guests in the hotel.

'I've not seen you in traditional dress before.' I say as I approach my friends and kiss each of them on the cheek. 'You look absolutely stunning. You too Lorna. I love that shade of purple. It goes so well with your grey hair!'

'I thought about wearing this outfit last night,' Adjavella confesses, 'Because a Boubou is often worn on special occasions, but I decided I would save it for Tilly's farewell today.'

'And she would have really appreciated it.' Lorna adds. 'Clothilde and I spent hours at the market as young teenagers, choosing fabrics for our dresses. Tell me about your headscarf, there must be a real knack to fixing it in place.'

'We're taught to wrap the moussor from a young age. We practice on each other, and on ourselves. They're a very individual and expressive part of our outfits.'

I feel a little underdressed next to these two, but I'm happy with the coral sundress I've chosen. Mam always liked orange and pink, and this dress combines the two. I've gone for a pair of white sandals on my feet, and of course I have Da's locket around my neck.

I'm also carrying a bright yellow cotton shoulder bag. It's not the most elegant of accessories, but I needed something big enough for the urn. If Adjavella has a purse, it's hidden within the folds of her outfit, and Lorna is clutching a very elegant leather handbag, which I know contains the handwritten tribute that she's been agonising over.

We turn into the car park and pull up beside Philippe's car. Lorna joins Simone on the back seat of their onward transport - up close the quadbike looks very unstable. I wonder at the wisdom of my suggestion. However,

Philippe is there waiting, ready to drive them the few hundred metres to the cliff edge, and they are both determined to make the trip.

Adjavella and I set off on foot along the sandy track. A few grasses have managed to take hold, but this harsh, wind-blown environment is not supportive of much vegetation.

I can see Fabienne and her daughters up ahead, and off to the left, as the track curves, I can see Odile as she walks along chatting to Erwan, fighting with her long hair, which is flowing horizontally in the offshore wind.

As we reach the cliff top the ground cover changes. Now, it is covered in what appears to be a carpet of pale-green sea broccoli. Seagulls are circling above us, and away to my right, I can see a small ruin on the furthest headland. It's a very remote location for any dwelling, and I wonder why it was built.

The coastline at this point is dramatic, with harsh cliffs of dark rock plunging down to a churning sea, but I can't see any sign of the arch. However, Philippe has stopped the quadbike on the next headland, so I assume he is at our destination.

I understand now why Simone didn't bring me here on my last visit. It's quite a way for anyone who is at all infirm, and this wind is starting to pick up. I'm genuinely worried that we may have to cancel, for fear of being blown off the cliff.

As we catch up with the others, I see that a small wooden barrier has been erected at ankle height, to discourage visitors from standing too close to the edge. I assume that this must be the viewing point.

I walk around behind the quadbike so that I can look back the way that I have come, and there below me is a huge arch, eroded from the cliff by the waves. From this angle it looks similar in size to the monumental arches in London and Paris but carved by nature rather than patriotic sculptors.

This is far more impressive than I had expected.

Odile is wrestling with the wind as she spreads a blanket on the ground and pins it down with the aid of a cool box holding some champagne. Philippe adds a couple of directors chairs for Lorna and Simone, and Rozenn and Nolwenn quickly sit on the other end of the blanket to keep it in place. Adjavella and I join them.

Luckily, although it's windy, it's not cold. With all of us huddled together on the blanket we should be able to hear each other speak.

Clothilde - 1958

Clothilde is up on the headland. The hem of her wedding dress has gone from pristine white to dirty yellow, but she doesn't care at all. They've been playing in the waves, dancing in the sand, singing songs and sharing stories. The party is still going on down on the beach, but she has climbed back up to check on the horses and have five minutes to herself.

She turns to look back down at the beach, and sees that James is also taking a moment. He's heading towards the arch. The tide has finally dropped low enough for him to walk through and out the other side.

Two nesting seagulls are defending their territory up here on the cliff, amongst the indefatigable coastal vegetation. Clothilde wonders about the place where she and James are going to create *their* nest. He speaks with such passion about the mainland coast near the Isle of Arran, but she has no idea what it will be like. Not as dramatic as here, he says.

The enormity of this move has just struck her. In four days, she will be leaving this peninsula forever. Her past has consistently undermined her present. She is still convinced that the only way to begin married life with hope for a solid future, is to leave France behind for good.

Her aunts say that her decision is forcing her to experience even more loss. They can't understand why she wants to go through it again. They don't understand the difference. This time, she is the one who is leaving. She will be the one never to return.

As a result, she can have a fresh start with no looking back. No yearning for France. No magnetic pull to somewhere she is not wanted. No wondering, why her family members have not written, or whether they are ill.

No more feelings like the ones she's had today, because the Stewarts are not here. She knows they were desperate to come, but the decision was out of their control. A smallpox outbreak placed their village in quarantine, and they were unable to travel.

Her mind understands the situation, but her heart does not. For over a decade, she had longed for their connections to be restored, and she'd finally allowed herself an expectation of happiness on her wedding day.

There is absolutely nothing like the pain of dashed hopes.

To remain in contact with everyone here in France would give each of them this same power to disappoint and hurt her, for years to come. If her future is just James and any children that they may have, then it will be easier for her to control the pain.

The day that she sets foot in Britain can be the day that Tilde MacLeod is born, and the start of a life of pure happiness.

Isla - 2019

We decide that Lorna should start our sharing of memories, as she knew Mam first. Simone will follow, with a short contribution from me about our time in Scotland as a family. Adjavella will speak last, about Mam's final year, before I scatter the ashes.

Lorna holds her piece of paper tightly as it flaps in the wind, and speaks with a determination to honour her friend, despite her emotion.

'The very first day Clothilde and I met, she was four, and I was six, and Paris had just fallen to the Nazis.'

Lorna - 1940

Lorna is unsure why she is wearing her best dress - as she is standing beside her father outside their next-door neighbours' house. He knocks, which is also something they would never normally do. They usually just open the door and go straight in, calling out if no one's in the kitchen.

Chloe opens the door and very formally invites them inside. There, in the corner of the kitchen, is a little girl with blonde, shoulder-length hair. She is wearing a smock-dress and sturdy lace up shoes. She looks scared and is firmly clutching the hand of a very beautiful woman, who must be her mother.

'Lorna, I would like you to meet my granddaughter Clothilde. She has come to live with us, and it would be nice if you could become friends.'

Chloe - 1940

Chloe is a little unsure whether this plan will work. There is such a vast difference in size and confidence between the two girls. Clothilde has barely said a word to anyone since she arrived. She simply follows her mother around, holding onto the edge of her skirt. Even here in the kitchen, she has only swapped the skirt-edge for her mother's hand.

Chloe is therefore greatly relieved, when Lorna strides purposefully across the room, takes Clothilde's free hand, and says,

'Come with me. I want to show you the piglets.'

Isla - 2019

I watch as an indulgent smile spreads across Lorna's face.

'From the moment she saw those piglets she looked to me for adventure, and we got into endless trouble together from that day onwards.'

Everyone chuckles at the thought of these two little wartime tearaways.

'Clothilde's adventurous spirit was a quality that I was lucky to see. Sadly, it was a characteristic that was later overwhelmed, by the anxieties that came with her mother's disappearance and her grandfather's death.' Lorna swallows hard. 'But I think it was a resurgence of this spirit, which helped her to connect with James and choose a life in a country far from everyone she knew.'

I look around me and we are all nodding our agreement.

'Although I was devastated when we were quarantined, and I was unable to attend Clothilde's wedding, I remember clearly how overjoyed I was the day that I received the invitation. As, during the two years when she and James were estranged, I had thought that fear had beaten her once again.'

Lorna grips her paper tightly in the wind.

'1956 was a marvellous year. I received several wonderful letters, in which she told me how she had fallen for James, but not everyone here would approve, so they were keeping their relationship a secret. I was so intrigued to know what it was about him that they wouldn't like and thrilled to be the keeper of her secret. However, in 1957 my joy turned to sadness, as it became clear that she had pushed James away, to avoid being hurt by his departure.'

Clothilde - 1956

Clothilde has the house to herself, so she is sitting at the kitchen table, writing to Lorna.

My dear friend,
I wish you were here. I feel as though, once again, my life is over. I returned last week from a trip with Neven to Sarzeau, and as I had predicted, James was gone.
Simone insists that he came looking for me, and that he was distraught to find me absent. But he was always going to leave.
Meeting James was the best thing that's ever happened to me, and our relationship was the most mature connection that I've had with a man, but I'm unconvinced that human relationships are something that I should pursue.
They are just too painful.
I've been cycling every day to the chapel, and I have gained a lot of comfort from the peace and solitude that I find there. I know this will surprise you, but I truly think that my future may lie within the church.
I hope that Rory and Dominique are keeping well and that your teaching is bringing you fulfilment.
Your loving friend
Clothilde.

Isla - 2019

Lorna clears her throat.

'The one thing that I know about my beautiful friend, is that when she did love, she loved deeply, and she honoured that love long after the physical person was gone. I spent hours helping her tend the rose bushes that she had planted in memory of her parents and her grandparents, and today, I've brought with me some dried petals that come from those very same plants. So, for Clothilde, and for everyone she loved and who loved her, I scatter them to the wind.'

With these unexpected and beautiful words, Lorna rises from her chair, reaches into her handbag and in one smooth movement releases a cloud of coloured petals into the wind. They swirl around our heads for a moment and are then whisked out to sea to dance with the gulls and the spray from the waves.

I swallow multiple times as the tears gush down my face and I think my heart will burst. I turn to Simone and see that she too is crying. I leave a moments silence for us all to reflect before inviting her to speak.

'As the eldest here, and Clothilde's aunt, it might have been supposed that I would have met her first, but life during the 1930s was much more local than people brought up in this globalised world, may realise.'

She turns to Nolwenn and Rozenn as she says this.

'I idolised her father Henri - my much older brother - and eagerly anticipated his every visit. So, you can imagine how excited I was, when I heard that he had had a baby daughter. I was also very proud, that I was going to become an aunt at the age of eight.'

'I remember the same feeling when I was thirteen.' Odile interrupts, smiling indulgently at Philippe.

'In those days, people with small babies rarely made unnecessary journeys, and neither my sister Renée, nor I, were considered old enough to travel to Paris to meet Clothilde.

Unfortunately, their eagerly awaited first visit to us, here in Brittany, was cancelled by the outbreak of war. The resulting separation was so much longer than any of us ever expected.'

I can see that this is an emotional topic for Simone, and I reach up to where her hand is resting on the wooden arm of her chair and give it a squeeze. She looks down at me as she continues.

'The joy I felt when she moved here to join us was only tempered by my sorrow that we didn't have the space for her to live with us at the farm. She was truly happy there amongst the animals. You only had to watch her grooming a horse or feeding the chickens to see the anxiety drop away from her face, and the haunted look disappear from her eyes.'

Tears are now running freely down the faces of the two elderly women, who had been so close to Mam through this period, and judging that it may be time to speak myself, I wriggle around to sit on my knees.

'It must have hurt each of you deeply when Mam chose to leave you behind, but if there is one positive thing to have come from that decision, it is that I don't recognise the haunted look that Simone has just described.

By moving to Scotland, and starting a new life as Tilly MacLeod, Mam did find the peace that she was looking for. At least most of the time. I have to admit that I myself, was probably the cause of a resurgence of anxiety and anguish in her life, when, in my ignorance of her past, I chose to base my life in Germany.'

I swallow deeply. This is harder than I'd thought.

'We had many happy times, full of laughter, in coastal areas of Scotland that are not so different from here. And the depth of her relationship with Da is something that most couples only strive for.'

Tilly - 1969

Tilly is sitting on the jetty, her toes dangling in the water of the loch, watching James and Isla playing in the shallows. James is trying to teach Isla to swim, but she's much more interested in scooping up large handfuls of water to throw at him.

It brings back wonderful memories of days at Plage de Kerbougnec, and Plage du Conguel, when James was so patient as she faced her fear of the water, and where she grew to love the feeling of his hands on her body, and the sound of his laugh.

It is utterly astonishing that a freak storm at sea can have been responsible for bringing her not only a loyal, dependable, handsome husband, but also a beautiful gem of a daughter.

What she has sacrificed in exchange is so painful that only golden moments such as these are powerful enough to bring thoughts of her homeland to the surface, where they can sneak past her determination to forget.

The peace of mind, which has come with restarting her life here in Scotland, has been a gift that would be indescribable, to anyone unfamiliar with inner torment and anxiety.

She has never known calm like it, and although she still experiences occasional, intense episodes of distress, they are few and far between. Her daily life has had an ease about it, unknown during her years in France. This change has been an important part of the process, by which she is developing the strength to be a mother.

There are days when she wonders how mothers behave, and as Isla now approaches the age at which Tilly's own mother disappeared, she can feel her anxieties growing.

But James is a wonderful father, and an even better husband, and he can sense when her anxieties are spiralling out of control.

At these moments, he either takes Isla out of the house, so that Tilly can have some space to collect herself, or if it's late at night, he holds Tilly tight, as they lie together in bed, speaking softly into her ear, and reminding her that their little family is safe, and that he loves her.

Isla - 2019

Adjavella sits up on her knees to speak, her hands resting evenly on her thighs.

'I met Tilly at a moment of crisis. James had just died, and she was so distraught and confused that her thoughts and emotions leapt to the time and place where the two of them met, here in France with all of you.

However, as she had reverted to speaking in French, this isolated her from the people in Scotland who were caring for her, and also from Isla, who at that time spoke no French - something that is now rather hard to believe.' She looks across at me with a crinkly, indulgent smile.

'The months that I had with Tilly in Scotland, acting as her translator, were absolutely unique in my life. I have cared for many people, but never have I met a person with such a strong life force. It battled through the confusion of her dementia, as she tried to make sense of the world around her and shone vividly as she told me of the people she had loved.

I believe it also showed itself in the utter determination of her healthy brain to keep the secret of her early years, in order that the life she had created with James could be preserved. Her brain fought itself for hours in front of me, as she would start to speak a train of thought, and then silence herself. It was only at the very end that I came to understand the battle that she'd fought.

And of course, through the mother, I met the daughter. I remember so clearly the first day that I met Isla. She was absolutely convinced that I must be lying about her mother's language skills.'

She glances my way, and all I can do is look sheepish.

'Luckily we got over that, and as you can see, we have become firm friends, forming an excellent team, to unravel the puzzle of Tilly's life, and find our way to the truth.'

I reach forward and place my hand on top of hers, for a moment of silence, until she continues.

'I am immensely grateful to have known Tilly, for that is the name by which I knew her, and thankful that I can be here with all of you, to say goodbye.'

Taking this as my cue, I stand up for my next contribution.

'I think now, it is time that I head down to the beach. Any of you who would like to join me, please make your way there now. I can see that the path is very steep, so please don't feel obliged. The tide is far enough out that you will be able to see everything from here.'

I'm glad that Mam's ashes are in the shoulder bag, as I need both hands free to balance myself on the way down.

Once I reach the beach, I remove my sandals, and tuck the hem of my dress up into my underwear. I take the urn from the bag and make my way to the sea. The waves are choppy, but not too large, so there is little chance of me being swept out to sea, as I step into the icy cold water of the Atlantic.

Fabienne is standing just behind, and to one side of me on the beach. I can feel her unspoken support, and I need it, because suddenly, I'm unable to go through with this.

'I've got this wrong. What am I doing? She should be with Da! Everything we've heard today is about how much they loved each other, and never wanted to be apart.'

Fabienne hoists up her own dress and wades in beside me.

'Isla, you don't have to worry about that. You showed me where you scattered James's ashes. The waters of the Firth of Clyde eventually flow out into the Atlantic, so there is nothing keeping them apart. James found her here once, and he will do so again.'

And so, with my newfound family all around me, I return Mam to the location where she got married, the region where she grew up, and the country of her birth.

Acknowledgements

The Lost Life of Tilly MacLeod is a multi-media fundraising and awareness project for dementia. It has many strands that have been developed with the help of a generous and compassionate group of people. The creation of this novel has been possible thanks to friends and family who have given me support and encouragement, and a marvellous group of writing professionals, and fellow attendees connected with The RNA New Writers' Scheme and Writers' Weekend who offered help and advice at conferences, in 1:1 sessions, and on courses. I would particularly like to thank Alison May, Julia Williams and Lily Fehim for their in-depth work on the manuscript.